Immigrants and Social Work: Thinking Beyond the Borders of the United States

Immigrants and Social Work: Thinking Beyond the Borders of the United States has been co-published simultaneously as *Journal of Immigrant & Refugee Services*, Volume 2, Numbers 1/2 2004.

Immigrants and Social Work: Thinking Beyond the Borders of the United States

Diane Drachman, PhD
Ana Paulino, EdD
Editors

Immigrants and Social Work: Thinking Beyond the Borders of the United States has been co-published simultaneously as *Journal of Immigrant & Refugee Services*, Volume 2, Numbers 1/2 2004.

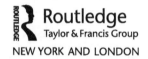

Routledge
Taylor & Francis Group
NEW YORK AND LONDON

First published by
The Haworth Press, Inc.
10 Alice Street
Binghamton, N Y 13904-1580

This edition published 2011 by Routledge

Routledge
Taylor & Francis Group
711 Third Avenue
New York, NY 10017

Routledge
Taylor & Francis Group
2 Park Square, Milton Park
Abingdon, Oxon OX14 4RN

Immigrants and Social Work: Thinking Beyond the Borders of the United States has been co-published simultaneously as *Journal of Immigrant & Refugee Services*, Volume 2, Numbers 1/2 2004.

The development, preparation, and publication of this work has been undertaken with great care. However, the publisher, employees, editors, and agents of The Haworth Press and all imprints of The Haworth Press, Inc. including The Haworth Medical Press® and Pharmaceutical Products Press®, are not responsible for any errors contained herein or for consequences that may ensue from use of materials or information contained in this work. Opinions expressed by the author(s) are not necessarily those of The Haworth Press, Inc. With regard to case studies, identities and circumstances of individuals discussed herein have been changed to protect confidentiality. Any resemblance to actual persons, living or dead, is entirely coincidental.

The Haworth Press, Inc., 10 Alice Street, Binghamton, NY 13904-1580 USA

Cover design by Jennifer Gaska

Library of Congress Cataloging-in-Publication Data
Immigrants and social work: thinking beyond the borders of the United States / Diane Drachman, Ana Paulino.
      p. cm.
   "Co-published simultaneously as Journal of Immigrant & Refugee Services, Volume 2, Numbers 1/2 2004.
   Includes bibliographical references and index.
   ISBN 0-7890-1998-1 (hard cover : alk. paper)–ISBN 0-7890-1999-X (soft cover : alk. paper)
      1. Social work with immigrants–United States. 2. Return migration. 3. Transnationalism.
I. Paulino, Ana. II. Journal of immigrant & refugee services (Online) III. Title.
HV4011.U5D72 2004
362.8–dc22   2004009662

ABOUT THE EDITORS

Diane Drachman, PhD, is Associate Professor at the University of Connecticut School of Social Work. The grants she received from the National Institute of Mental Health and the Office of Refugee Resettlement have enabled her to develop curriculum on social work practice with immigrant and refugee populations; to work with and publish on varied immigrant and refugee groups; and to develop a generic framework aimed at understanding immigrant and refugee populations as well as understanding the individual or family in the context of migration. Her recent publications synthesize social work knowledge with immigration law, immigration history and migration studies. She teaches courses on direct practice with individuals and families and social work practice with immigrants and refugees. As a practitioner, she has worked in many regions of the United States in public welfare settings, family and children's service agencies, and community mental health organizations.

Ana Paulino, EdD, is Associate Professor at Hunter College School of Social Work, City University of New York. She serves as a consulting editor for the *Journal of Teaching in Social Work* and is a former consulting editor for the *Journal of Multicultural Social Work*. Dr. Paulino is a Consultant for private and governmental mental health agencies and has extensive experience in child welfare, family services, health, and mental health. She is a member of various community and professional Advisory Boards. She is a former recipient of several training grants from the state and city government for programs focusing on cultural competence, child welfare, and mental health issues. Her research and writing have focused on the areas of immigration, Dominican families in the United States, death and dying, spirituality, and community mental health. She teaches in the area of Social Casework, Social Work Practice with Families, Clinical Casework Practice with Children, Social Work Practice in School Settings, and Human Behavior & the Social Environment. She serves as chairperson for Children, Youth, and Families Area of Specialization.

Immigrants and Social Work: Thinking Beyond the Borders of the United States

CONTENTS

Foreword

The American profession of social work developed largely around the provision of services to immigrants. The writings of early pioneers in various fields of practice tell us of the importance of immigrant status. Charles Loring Brace, a founder of foster care headed the chapters in his book, "The Dangerous Classes of New York City and Twenty Years Work Among Them," according to the national origins of the children whose characteristics he described. Mary Richmond in her research reports to the Russell Sage Foundation on Charity Organization Societies' work among families similarly identified the groups served by the country of origin. In Jane Addams, *Twenty Years at Hull House,* she tells of the intense concentration of settlement house work among immigrants and ethnic enclaves. A consistent goal of these diverse social work efforts was the achievement of acculturation of the immigrants and their eventual assimilation into mainstream America. Given the enormous barriers of distance and expense, most of these immigrants were unlikely to maintain close and consistent ties to their homelands.

Twentieth century social work, while following this traditional course, was evolving at the same time that the patterns of immigration were becoming increasingly diverse and complex. The evolving United States immigration laws and policies added to this complexity with their Byzantine array of multiple economic and political motivations. The reasons for migration and the conditions of the countries of origin varied greatly as did the accompanying experiences of the immigrants themselves. In previous work, Drachman and her colleagues have given the profession valuable directives for the adaptation of social work intervention to these ever changing complexities. They have stressed the importance of understanding not

[Haworth co-indexing entry note]: "Foreword." Giovannoni, Jeanne M. Co-published simultaneously in *Journal of Immigrant & Refugee Services* (The Haworth Social Work Practice Press, an imprint of The Haworth Press) Vol. 2, No. 1/2, 2004, pp. xv-xvi; and: *Immigrants and Social Work: Thinking Beyond the Borders of the United States* (ed: Diane Drachman, and Ana Paulino) The Haworth Social Work Practice Press, an imprint of The Haworth Press, Inc., 2004, pp. xi-xii. Single or multiple copies of this article are available for a fee from The Haworth Document Delivery Service [1-800-HAWORTH, 9:00 a.m. - 5:00 p.m. (EST). E-mail address: docdelivery@haworthpress.com].

http://www.haworthpress.com/web/JIRS
Digital Object Identifier: 10.1300/J191v02n01

xi

just the experience of immigrating but also the varying pre-migration situations and experiences of these individuals. Beyond the common subjective experiences of migration, i.e., the pain of separation and the angst of newcomer adaptation–the pre-migratory experiences can strongly influence subsequent adjustments.

In this volume, Drachman and Paulino expand this perspective. The importance of the continuing relationship of immigrants to their homeland and their significant others there has now taken on new dimensions. For many, perhaps most, the concept of a linear model of acculturation and assimilation is no longer valid. This volume provides a rich resource, a new conceptualization of the variables involved in the diversity and complexities of the patterns of relationships to the country of origin which are the present day reality. Personal relationships are interdependent within enlarged family systems, transcending borders. Now, for many, travel and visitation are an integral part of life. Beyond this complexity there are myriad variations, both symbolic and instrumental, imposed by the political and economic ecologies in which these relationships are enmeshed.

This volume offers extraordinarily useful conceptual tools for understanding these complexities. Beyond the conceptual schemes which tie the contributors' works together, each of the individual pieces offers intriguing applications to the real world of practice, both micro and macro, and across several fields of practice as well as insightful suggestions for future research.

The work is crucially timely. For any who have had doubts that globalization is upon us, reading this volume will dispel any such doubts. This volume should prove to be genuinely helpful to the profession in adapting to this new and challenging environment, the environment that constitutes the life space of a longstanding social work clientele.

Jeanne M. Giovannoni, PhD
Professor Emerita of Social Welfare
University of California, Los Angeles

Introduction:
Thinking Beyond United States' Borders

Diane Drachman
Ana Paulino

SUMMARY. The United States social work literature on immigrants and immigration emphasizes one part of the migration process–the experiences of immigrants in this country. However, experiences in the country of origin that lead to emigration receive limited attention. Knowledge of the latter ultimately provides a context for understanding the immigration experience. This introduction, Thinking Beyond United States' Borders, presents the underlying ideas that provide the foundation for the discussions in this volume. It focuses on the interconnectedness between immigrants' country of origin and destination. Thus, a two-country perspective is embedded in this discussion and in the articles that follow. *[Article copies available for a fee from The Haworth Document Delivery Service: 1-800-HAWORTH. E-mail address: <docdelivery@haworthpress.com> Website: <http://www.HaworthPress.com> © 2004 by The Haworth Press, Inc. All rights reserved.]*

Diane Drachman, PhD, is Associate Professor, University of Connecticut School of Social Work.

Ana Paulino, EdD, is Associate Professor and Chair, Children, Youth, and Families Field of Practice/Specialization, Hunter College School of Social Work.

[Haworth co-indexing entry note]: "Introduction: Thinking Beyond United States' Borders." Drachman, Diane, and Ana Paulino. Co-published simultaneously in *Journal of Immigrant & Refugee Services* (The Haworth Social Work Practice Press, an imprint of The Haworth Press) Vol. 2, No. 1/2, 2004, pp. 1-9; and: *Immigrants and Social Work: Thinking Beyond the Borders of the United States* (ed: Diane Drachman, and Ana Paulino) The Haworth Social Work Practice Press, an imprint of The Haworth Press, Inc., 2004, pp. 1-9. Single or multiple copies of this article are available for a fee from The Haworth Document Delivery Service [1-800-HAWORTH, 9:00 a.m. - 5:00 p.m. (EST). E-mail address: docdelivery@haworthpress.com].

http://www.haworthpress.com/web/JIRS
© 2004 by The Haworth Press, Inc. All rights reserved.
Digital Object Identifier: 10.1300/J191v02n01_01

1

KEYWORDS. Social work, immigration, immigrants, return migration, transnationalism

Since 1965, the foreign-born population in the United States has been arriving from countries in Asia, Central America, the Caribbean, Africa, Eastern Europe and the Middle East. Like immigrants who arrived in previous waves, many have adapted well and made significant contributions to their new land. The process of migration, however, includes multiple stresses such as leaving one's family, friends, community and homeland. Upon arrival in the new country, immigrants need to obtain housing and employment, secure education for their children, learn a new language and ultimately become familiar with the ways of thinking and behaving of the people in their new land. These circumstances can be debilitating and render the population vulnerable and at risk for social, psychological, health, economic, legal, housing and employment problems.

Immigrants and refugees have been seen by social workers in the varied service settings in which they work such as community agencies, health and mental health organizations, schools, institutions in the welfare and justice systems, and in the work place. To understand their experiences, consideration of both emigration and immigration is necessary. According to the classical explanation of population movements, migration is the result of push and pull forces of sending and receiving countries. This explanation assumes that emigration and immigration are parts of a unitary process. Push forces from the country of origin commonly include political upheavals, severe economic circumstances, limited educational opportunity and social problems, such as persecution or discriminatory practices against an individual or group. Pull forces in the receiving country are generally economic, social or educational as immigrants anticipate better opportunities in these areas of life in their new country.

The United States' (U.S.) social work literature on immigrants and immigration, however, emphasizes one part of the migration process–the experiences of immigrants in this country. It focuses on specific groups such as immigrants from Asia, the Caribbean, Eastern Europe and Latinos. Cultural phenomena and family issues are also examined. Although these issues are important for understanding immigrant populations and providing services to them, this emphasis by-passes a significant dimension of the migration process–i.e., experiences associated with emigration. Thus, occurrences in the country of origin such as the departure experiences which can be abrupt, violent, or involve a long wait prior to leaving, decisions regarding who should leave and who would be left behind, community and family supports for emigration (or lack thereof), economic, social and political factors surrounding emigration, expectations for life in the new land and the multiple stresses unique to this phase of migration receive scant attention. Knowledge of the above would not only broaden social work understanding of the migratory process, it would also provide a context for understanding the immigration experience.

Historical and sociological analyses have widened and modified our understanding of the influences on migration beyond the macro push-pull forces of the classical explanation (Yans-McLaughlin, 1990; Tilly, 1990). These explanations of emigration and immigration incorporate notions of support networks, communities, and families in both sending and receiving countries. They discuss their influence on decisions to migrate, the point of destination, and the degree of adaptation to the new country. They also emphasize linkages between support networks in both sending and receiving countries (Tilly, 1990). For example, support networks in the old country that are connected to networks in the new country may enable recent immigrants to secure housing, employment, or other needed services.

Network structures also facilitate an understanding of a recent phenomenon in migration: transnationalism. Transnationalism refers to migrating populations whose networks, activities, and patterns of life encompass both home and host countries (Glick-Schiller, Basch, Blanc Szanton, 1992; Charles, 1992; Wiltshire, 1992). Transnational immigrants are therefore individuals whose lives and networks cut across national boundaries and whose social fields exist in two countries.

Many recent arrivals from Mexico, Guatemala, India, Pakistan, Africa, and the Caribbean are transnational immigrants. They often return to their home country for visits. Some return for long periods. Many send remittances to family members. Their contacts with families in the home country may involve them in decision making on health care or the education of children. While visiting, they may take part in political, social or religious activities. Concurrently, these immigrants are involved with their U.S. families. They are involved in the U.S. schools their children attend. They are involved in their places of employment, religious organizations, and ethnic communities in the U.S.

Networks of transnational immigrants benefit individuals and families in both sending and receiving countries. For example, family members in the home country often provide care for those children who do not migrate with their parent(s). Remittances from immigrants supplement the incomes of those who remain behind while networks in the new land commonly provide concrete help and social support for recent arrivals. Knowledge of the two-country experience, therefore, is necessary to adequately understand and provide services to the transnational immigrant population.

Recent attention is also paid to the phenomenon of return migration. Return migrants are persons who emigrate, live in a new country for years, and ultimately return to reside in their native land. In a recent description of Jamaican return migrants, the "returnees" indicate their fellow Jamaicans perceive them as nationals from the country to which they emigrated (John Small personal communication, 1999). Thus, they are viewed as either American, Canadian or English, etc., as they carry the behavior and ways of thinking of people from those countries. Although the "returnees" acknowledge they acquire some ways of thinking that are similar to the natives of those countries, they also view themselves both culturally and nationally as Jamaican. Ultimately they describe their experiences as "foreigners" in the country to which they emigrated and as "foreigners" in their homeland upon their return (John Small, personal communication, 1999). Similar to transnationals, it is necessary for social workers to understand the two-country experiences of the returnees in order to understand the phenomenon of return migration.

Changes in U.S. immigration law have a significant influence on the lives of many immigrants in the U.S. The changes also impact the families of immigrants who remain in the home countries. Furthermore, they create social and economic difficulties in the sending countries. Specifically, the 1996 Illegal Immigration Reform and Immigrant Responsibility Act (IIRIRA) establishes new provisions which result in the deportation of many individuals. Prior to the IIRIRA, immigrants who were issued an order of deportation had the right to appeal the order through judicial review. The new provisions, however, remove this right for classes of immigrants: persons convicted of an aggravated felony offense, persons convicted of an offense involving drugs, convictions for domestic violence, stalking, child abuse, child neglect, child abandonment, violations against immigration law and misdemeanors such as shoplifting (Medina, 1997). This feature of the law is also retroactive. Thus, an immigrant who committed an offense years ago is subject to immediate deportation despite the many years following the conviction when the individual raised a family, was consistently employed and led a productive life.

The deportation of many of these individuals has catastrophic affects on the families who remain in the U.S. Some families lose the income of the primary wage earner. Children are separated from a parent. Wives and husbands are separated from each other. Older adult parents are separated from their adult children.

The countries of origin where the deportees have been sent also experience difficulties due to the number of deportees they must absorb. Jamaica and other Caribbean countries, for example, do not have employment opportunities to accommodate the numbers that have arrived. Finally, the families who remained in the country of origin are negatively affected as they lose a significant source of their income since they no longer receive the remittances that were previously sent.

After the September 11, 2001 attack on the World Trade Center and the Pentagon, the U.S. responded legislatively with the passage of the Uniting and Strengthening America by Providing Appropriate Tools Required to Intercept and Obstruct Terrorism Act (USA Patriot Act). This legislation has a significant impact on immigrants living in the U.S. and their families living in their home countries. The law cedes to the Justice Department broad surveillance and detention powers over persons suspected of terrorism. Under the Act, a non-citizen can be detained for 7 days without being charged with either a criminal or immigration violation. If the non-citizen is charged with an immigration violation, he/she is subject to mandatory detention while removal proceedings are pending. The individual has no right to the evidence that supports the charge. The individual also has no right of counsel to contest the charge (Chang 2001; Liptak, 2003; Shenon, 2003). On the basis of secret information immigrants may therefore experience long detention stays without judicial review.

In the weeks and months after the September 11th attacks, 762 people were arrested. Although most of these individuals violated an immigration law such as visa overstay or illegal entry into the country, none were charged with a terror related crime (Lichtblau, 2003). According to an investigation of the Justice Department's actions, it was reported there was "little effort to distinguish legitimate terrorist suspects from others picked up in roundups of illegal immigrants" (Shenon, 2003). Many individuals were detained for a month or longer without being told why they were being held. Furthermore, detention centers routinely blocked efforts by detainees' families and lawyers to locate them (Liptak, 2003). Thus, families of the detainees living in the U.S. and those living in their home countries could not find or contact their detained relatives. Ultimately the lives of immigrants are influenced by the policies, circumstances and events that exist in both the sending and receiving countries.

To broaden social work knowledge in the area of migration, this volume focuses on the interconnectedness between immigrants' country of origin and destination. Thus, a two-country perspective is embedded in the analysis of the migration experience discussed by the authors in the volume. This focus facilitates thinking beyond a U.S. context when providing services to individuals, families and groups, designing and developing service programs, community organizing, policy analysis, political practice, and research.

The ideas described in the above section are illustrated in the qualitative research of Drs. Marquez and Padilla who describe and analyze the immigration stories of low income Mexican women living on both sides of the U.S./Mexico border. The study is framed within the view of migration as a process versus migration as an event. As the authors state, the life stories of the women provide a "snapshot along a continuum of processes that are involved in migration." Embedded in the work is the interrelationship between issues and events that occur in the country/region of origin with those that occur in the country or region of resettlement.

Drs. Humphreys and Haroutunian discuss the Armenian diaspora and the return of Armenian refugees (or children of refugees) from the diaspora to the new republic of Armenia. These individuals, who are citizens of other countries, returned to Armenia to assist displaced persons who survived a massive earthquake in the newly formed country. The development of voluntary social services and a school of social work in Armenia is in part the result of their contributions. The discussion ultimately illustrates the interconnection between peoples' native land and "new" land, and the interaction among institutions in the homeland and "new" land that emerge out of migration.

The historic and current connection between international social work and practice with immigrants and refugees presented by Dr. Healy assumes knowledge that extends beyond U.S. borders. The experiences of the transnational family whose members live in separate countries some times living apart for years and who often re-unify are examined within a dual lens of home and "host" countries. The remittances which immigrants send to families in the home country are also examined in the context of the sending and receiving countries.

The back and forth movement of individuals from the island of Puerto Rico to the U.S. mainland is examined by Dr. Acevedo under the concept of circular migration. Highlighted are the macro forces in the two lands that generate circular migration. The influence of this type of migration on family life and structure has implications for practice with this population as well as policy considerations.

The discussion of migration from the Dominican Republic presented by Dr. Hernández is examined within an historical context. Attention is paid to the historical interconnectedness of changing political, economic and social forces in both the sending country of the Dominican Republic and the receiving country of the United States. Thus a longitudinal view of the interconnectedness of two countries' policies regarding migration is presented.

Dr. Guzzetta explores the phenomenon of return migration, i.e., persons who return to their homeland after having lived in the country of destination for a significant period of time. Important questions regarding the definition of return migrants are raised. For example, are transnational and circular immigrants also return migrants? These definitional issues are relevant for social workers as it is likely that individuals and families' experiences associated with transnational and circular migration are different from each other and different from persons who return to their homeland as retirees.

The challenging experiences of undocumented Mexican immigrants when departing from their native country and the challenges they encounter in the receiving country of the U.S. are presented by Dr. Zuniga. The description of the two-country experiences, which are life threatening for some people, provides social workers with useful background information for assessment of individuals' mental health and social functioning. The economic factors of business cycles and labor needs and their influence on the lives of undocumented immigrants and their families in the sending country and in the receiving country of the U.S. are also examined. Useful practice approaches are discussed in the context of the above issues and in the context of U.S. policies that affect the undocumented immigrant population.

Dr. Chung and Ms. Samperi's discussion of the philosophy, design, and helping approach of a program that serves a Chinese immigrant population suffering from chronic mental illness illustrates the integration of an "East-West" mode of service delivery. The unique meaning and experience of emigration and the meaning of mental illness held by the Chinese immigrant clients and their families are incorporated in the helping milieu. Similarly, United States' views and ways of approaching mental "illness" are introduced. Thus, service delivery is rooted in the views of people from both the country of origin and destination. Finally, the discussions in this volume with their focus on sending and receiving countries are presented within different domains of social work. Policy analysis explains forces embedded in Puerto Rican and Dominican migration. Mental health issues that derive from the traumatic events experienced by undocumented Mexican immigrants are identified. The description of a cross national collaboration between educators in the U.S. and Armenia provide information on social work curriculum development. The discussion of return migration facilitates teaching and learning about a phase in the migration process. The migration experiences of women living in U.S./Mexico border towns obtained from qualitative research provide insights into the unique and individual stories of women in migration. In a discussion of international social work, we learn about the transnational family. Finally, a culturally consonant mode of service delivery is portrayed in the description of a program designed for Chinese immigrants.

REFERENCES

Chang, N. (2001). The U.S.A. Patriot Act. *Center for Constitutional Rights.* Retrieved September 18, 2002, from *http://ccr-ny.org/what'snew/usa* patriot act.

Charles, C.(1992). Transnationalism in the construct of Haitian migrants' racial categories of identity in New York City. In N. Glick-Schiller, L. Basch, & C. Blanc-Szanton (Eds.) *Towards a transnational perspective on migration: Race, class, ethnicity and nationalism reconsidered* (pp. 101-123). New York: New York Academy of Sciences.

Glick-Schiller, N., Basch, L., & Blanc-Szanton, C. (1992). Transnationalism: A new analytic framework for understanding migration. In N. Glick-Schiller, L. Basch, & C. Blanc-Szanton (Eds.) *Towards a transnational perspective on migration: Race, class, ethnicity and nationalism reconsidered* (pp. 1-24). New York: New York Academy of Sciences.

Lichtblau, E. (2003). U.S. report faults the roundup of illegal immigrants after 9/11. *New York Times,* June 3, PA1.

Liptak, A. (2003). For jailed immigrants a presumption of guilt. *New York Times,* June 3, PA18.

Medina, I. (1997). Judicial review–A nice thing? Article III, Separation of Powers and the Illegal Immigration Reform and Immigrant Responsibility Act of 1996. *Connecticut Law Review,* 29(4), 1525-1563. University of Connecticut School of Law.

Shenon, P. (2003). Report on U.S. antiterrorism law alleges violations of civil rights. *New York Times,* July 21, PA1.

Small, J. (1999). Personal communication.

Tilly, C. (1990). Transplanted networks. In V. Yans-McLaughlin (Ed.). *Immigration reconsidered: History, sociology and politics* (pp. 79-95). New York, New York: Oxford University Press.

Wiltshire, R. (1992). Implications of transnational migration for nationalism: The Caribbean example. In N. Glick-Schiller, L. Basch, & C. Blanc-Szanton (Eds.) *Towards a transnational perspective on migration: Race, class, ethnicity and national ism reconsidered* (pp. 175-188). New York: New York Academy of Science.

Yans-McLaughlin, V. (1990). Introduction. In V. Yans-McLaughlin (Ed.). *Immigration reconsidered: History, sociology and politics* (pp. 3-18). New York: Oxford University Press.

Immigration in the Life Histories of Women Living in the United States-Mexico Border Region

Raquel R. Marquez
Yolanda C. Padilla

SUMMARY. This paper focuses on the role that immigration plays in the lives of very low-income women living along the United States-Mexico border. Life here is distinct from that in any other part of the United States, due to the international, social, political, and economic interdependence that characterizes this region. Thus, from the perspective of migration as a social process, this "contact zone" can provide insight on migration issues that occur within a transborder context.

Raquel R. Marquez, PhD, is Assistant Professor, Department of Sociology, and Research Affiliate, the Hispanic Research Center and the Institute for Law Research, University of Texas at San Antonio.

Yolanda C. Padilla, PhD, MSSW, is Associate Professor, School of Social Work, and Research Affiliate, the Center for Mexican American Studies and the Population Research Center, University of Texas at Austin.

This study was part of a larger research project funded by the MacArthur Foundation to examine the life chances of women living in poverty along the United States-Mexico border region.

In addition to the cities of Brownsville, Texas and Matamoros, Tamaulipas, Mexico, the study included two other sister border cities, El Paso, Texas, and Juarez, Chihuahua, Mexico.

[Haworth co-indexing entry note]: "Immigration in the Life Histories of Women Living in the United States-Mexico Border Region." Marquez, Raquel R., and Yolanda C. Padilla. Co-published simultaneously in *Journal of Immigrant & Refugee Services* (The Haworth Social Work Practice Press, an imprint of The Haworth Press) Vol. 2, No. 1/2, 2004, pp. 11-30; and: *Immigrants and Social Work: Thinking Beyond the Borders of the United States* (ed: Diane Drachman, and Ana Paulino) The Haworth Social Work Practice Press, an imprint of The Haworth Press, Inc., 2004, pp. 11-30. Single or multiple copies of this article are available for a fee from The Haworth Document Delivery Service [1-800-HAWORTH, 9:00 a.m. - 5:00 p.m. (EST). E-mail address: docdelivery@haworthpress.com].

http://www.haworthpress.com/web/JIRS
Digital Object Identifier: 10.1300/J191v02n01_02

Based on life history interviews and focus groups with women living in two adjoining border cities, Brownsville, Texas and Matamoros, Tamaulipas, we observed the trajectories of women at two points of the migration course: (a) migration from the interior of Mexico to the northern border and (b) emigration across the international boundary to the United States. The study shows that although these women held expectations that migration would improve their lives and the lives of their families, their social and economic integration in the border region met with limited success. *[Article copies available for a fee from The Haworth Document Delivery Service: 1-800-HAWORTH. E-mail address: <docdelivery@haworthpress.com> Website: <http://www.HaworthPress.com>* © 2004 by The Haworth Press, Inc. All rights reserved.]*

KEYWORDS. Migration, immigration, transborder, United States-Mexico border, *maquiladoras, colonias,* life histories, poverty, women, Mexican Americans

Because Mexicans comprise by far the largest group of immigrants in the United States, there has been great interest in the dynamics of immigration in this population. As of 1980, Mexico became the leading source of immigrants to the United States, and in 1997 Mexicans comprised a full 27.5 percent of all immigrants to the United States (Schmidley & Gibson, 1999). This figure is about six times as large as the next highest-ranked country, the Philippines. Nevertheless, the study of Mexican immigration has been very fragmented, with an emphasis on the assimilation of immigrants once they are already living in this country (Baca-Zinn, 1998; Hondagneu-Sotelo, 1994; Portes, 1985). The full story of immigration is much richer than that, and all the more for Mexican immigrants to the United States, because of the geographic, social, and historical interconnections between the two countries (Marquez, 1998; Padilla, 1996). Exploring the lives of people along the international border of the United States and Mexico, who are at various stages of migration, presents a unique opportunity to observe a snapshot of the continuum within these migration processes (Drachman, 1992). We are then able to piece together migration stories, from the dreams of a search for a better life, to prior journeys within their native lands, to the process of arrival in the new country, and finally to the course of integration in the shadow of the homeland. Our research allowed us to follow women along multiple points in the continuum of the migration process, although the study revealed that this process did not always follow a linear trajectory, but rather that the road between destinations was often filled with obstacles and detours.

In order to grasp all the complexity of immigration as a process, rather than as an event, in this study we utilize life histories to uncover the immigration stories of people living on both sides of the US-Mexico border. Although at times driven by political reasons, Mexicans are above all economic immigrants (Bean et al., 1997; Hondagneu-Sotelo, 1994; Roberts & Escobar-Lapati, 1997). They come to the United States to improve their economic conditions, often driven by harsh realities of poverty in their country of origin (Bean et al., 1997; Roberts & Escobar-Lapati, 1997; Marquez, 1998). Relative to other immigrants and to native-born Mexican Americans, Mexican immigrants in the United States have very low educational, occupational, and income levels (Gelbard & Carter, 1997). Only 31 percent of Mexican immigrants have completed high school, only 6 percent are in professional or managerial occupations and 31 percent are in the laborer occupations, and 33.9 percent live below the poverty level, the highest rate of any other foreign-born population (Schmidley & Gibson, 1999). To capture the substance of the economic precariousness in the lives of immigrants, in this study we chose to focus on a population living in poverty. We further chose to hear the stories of families and households from the perspective of women, a perspective that has received less attention in the research on immigration. Although women's participation in migration has been viewed from the perspective of their role in the labor force, feminist theory conceptualizes the migration of Mexican women as a survival strategy (Gonzalez et al., 1995; Hondagneu-Sotelo, 1994). Thus, the focus on women allows us to more closely examine the effects of labor market trends on households and their concomitant strategies for survival in the face of disadvantage (González de la Rocha, 1994).

Until recently, research on Mexican immigration to the United States paid limited attention to women's participation in the migration process (Portes, 1985; Massey, 1986 &1987). The major contribution of recent research, which views women's migration in the context of household survival strategies, has been the study of the relationship between women's migration decisions and gender roles. According to Hondagneu-Sotelo in *Gendered Transitions: Mexican Experiences of Immigration*, women's immigration and settlement experience reflect gender relations that are "reflexively intertwined." In her study of immigrant women in California, she finds that the negotiation of immigration and settlement helps immigrants reconstruct their gender relations within their families and in their new communities (Hondagneu-Sotelo, 1994). Similarly, sociologist Curry Rodriguez finds a strong relationship between female labor migration and the redefinition of traditional gender responsibilities (Curry Rodriguez, 1988). Finally, studies of female migration on the US-Mexico border show that the movement across the border by men is closely related to work, while women's travel is more frequently associated with family (Gonzalez et al., 1995). Thus, women's migration experiences are motivated by traditional concerns for family economic roles in their new environments.

BACKGROUND

The boundary that separates the United States and Mexico extends some 2000 miles from California to Texas. Yet, rather than separating the two countries, in many ways it functions as a connection between interdependent communities on each side of the border forming a distinct region. Therefore, the borderlands encompasses two peoples, two countries, two languages and everything that falls in between, and here at the border these two halves meet and interact as one, or a transborder region. Fundamental to this idea are the everyday interactions which bridge the two sides; interactions that routinely include the norms, practices, and family ties from both sides of the border. Through these links, the region functions as a transnational community for the actors in this daily drama (D'Antonio, 1965; Price, 1969; Marquez, 1998; Martinez, 1986).

Border communities also share other less desirable factors, such as a sometime harsh tropical climate, social and political isolation within their own countries, and the brunt force of a divisive, international boundary (Marquez, 1998; Padilla, Lein & Cruz, 1999). An important imbalance occurs at the economic level, because the US' side lacks the high level of economic activity exhibited by Northern Mexican border cities (Escobar & Roberts, 1998; Marquez, 1998). As a result of this economic environment, Northern Mexican border towns are frequent points of destination for Mexican migrants in search of work and a better life for their families (Roberts & Escobar-Lapati, 1997; Escobar & Roberts, 1998; Marquez, 1998).

When discussing the relevance of the economic development of South Texas to immigration, it is always important to return to the issue of poverty. The interrelationship of immigration, economic development, and poverty is key to understanding the current economic and social relations of the region. Historically, work opportunities for Mexican American women were available primarily in factories and sometimes in agricultural, industries that increased their profits through the labor of poor and unskilled women (Marquez, 1995). Issues of language and education along with racial and ethnic barriers created a segmented and stratified labor force that forced Mexican women to the bottom of the social and economic ladder and kept them in poverty (Ledesma, 1992). The region's industrial development was successful by taking advantage of the availability of an abundant and cheap labor force. Thus, the region's current impoverished conditions have a long history of exploitation (Marquez, 1995). This is the historical legacy that embraces immigrant women who settle in South Texas.

Today, various points along the United States-Mexico borderlands are the most frequent place of destination for those who come from the interior of Mexico (Roberts & Escobar-Lapati, 1997; Escobar & Roberts, 1998). From the macro-level, global events, such as the integration of capital-intensive industrialization into Latin American economies, have increased inequality in countries like Mexico (Marrujo, 1995; Escobar & Roberts, 1998). Furthermore, gender inequality for Mexican women has been heightened by urbanization and industrialization, key issues that have spurred women's migration from Mexico's interior to the borderlands. Women move to the border seeking to improve their lives, but conditions in border cities make the transition difficult. On the Mexican side of the border, many women find work in *maquiladoras*, assembly-line industrial plants that are well known for exploitative working conditions that have widespread affects on their dominant female labor force (Marquez, 1998; Marrujo, 1995; Pena, 1997). Today's larger *maquiladoras* are primarily owned by foreign companies and are situated along sister city points like Matamoros and Brownsville (Marrujo, 1995; Escobar & Roberts, 1998). Pay at these plants is relatively good by Mexican standards, but the high costs at the border offset the few gains the women earn. Poverty runs high where newcomers settle, and the region's infrastructure struggles to meet the demands of a constant influx of arrivals (Roberts & Escobar-Lapati, 1997; Escobar & Roberts, 1998; Marquez, 1998). Often, migrating to the US side of the border is the next step for these women. What women who settle on the US side find, however, are that they face similar conditions as they attempt to integrate into their new communities.

METHODOLOGY

To learn more about how the effects of transnational forces in the United States-Mexico border region are expressed in the lives of individuals and families, we interviewed women living on adjacent cities of the international boundary. A total of 28 women were interviewed: 12 women living on the US side of the Border, in Brownsville, Texas, and 16 women living on the Mexican side, in Matamoros, Tamaulipas. This area was selected because it is a major border-crossing site, and because the Brownsville region is considered one of the poorest areas of the United States (Maril, 1989; Marquez, 1998; Padilla, Lein & Cruz, 1999; Texas Comptroller, 1998). Data were obtained using two methods, oral life histories and focus groups. Oral histories were gathered for a total of 15 women, 8 in Brownsville and 7 in Matamoros. Another 13 women participated in focus groups conducted in each city, 4 in Brownsville and 9 in Matamoros.

A life history is "a retrospective account by an individual of his life in whole or part, in written or oral form, that has been elicited or prompted by another person" (Watson & Watson, 1985, p. 2). A detailed life history follows an individual's life course. This method of research provides an in-depth understanding essential to qualitative research (Hondagneu-Sotelo, 1994; Marquez, 1998; Sherraden & Barrera, 1995; Zavella, 1993). Life histories provide rich information through their open-ended format; information that the researcher had not necessarily set out to explore (Barahona, 1985; Langness, 1981). Focus group interviews complement individual-level interviews by providing an opportunity for respondents to discuss their ideas with each other (Reviere et al., 1996).

The life histories covered the period between the times that each woman first considered migration up until the day she was interviewed. During the interviews each woman outlined her life trajectory during this time frame focusing on family and work events related to her migration experience. Most interviews were conducted in the respondents' homes and ranged from 1 1/2 to 2 1/2 hours. In addition to the individual interviews, focus group interviews covered issues related to the perspectives of the respondents concerning life chances on the United States-Mexico border. The majority of the interviews were conducted in Spanish although some of the Brownsville interviews were done in English and in the Brownsville focus group participants switched back and forth between languages, a common practice among US border residents.

In Brownsville, women who had migrated to the United States from Mexico were interviewed. The research data was collected from three groups of immigrant women: women who were originally from the Mexican border region, women who had migrated from the interior of Mexico prior to migrating to the United States, and women who had recently crossed into the United States. In order to obtain a bi-national perspective on US' immigration dynamics, women whose internal Mexican migration had brought them to the border region and who at the time of the interview lived in Matamoros were also interviewed. In the Matamoros setting, the group included long-term settlers as well as more recently arrived internal migrants. Women in both cities were recruited from several pre-selected high poverty areas. In Brownsville, all respondents lived in very poor neighborhoods which are unique to the Texas Mexico border region and which are known as *colonias* (see Teaching Point box). Respondents were located using a snowball technique and through introductions by local key informants and other contacts and by knocking on neighborhood doors. Tables 1 and 2 provide descriptive information on the age, marital status, birthplace, and occupation of each of the women who were interviewed individually in Matamoros and Brownsville, respectively. The women who were recruited to participate in the focus groups closely matched these profiles. However, an individual questionnaire was not administered to focus group participants.

EXPECTATIONS FOR A NEW LIFE: INTERNAL MIGRATION TO THE NORTHERN MEXICO BORDER

The women we interviewed in Matamoros migrated to northern Mexico from all parts of Mexico with the belief that here they would find

TABLE 1. Characteristics of Women Interviewed in Matamoros

Name[a]	Age	Marital Status	Birthplace	Occupation
Teresa	27	Single	Ciudad Mante, Tamaulipas	Accountant, custom shipping company
Graciela	26	Separated (no children)	Papantla, Veracruz	Maquila, copper wiring welder
Celia	26	Single	Tamazunchale, San Luis Potosi	Maquila, computer systems
Luisa	29	Married (husband not living with her)	Monterrey, Nuevo Leon	Maquila, auto parts assembly
Lupe	24	Single	Tampico, Tamaulipas	Assistant researcher
Rosario	49	Single mother	San Luis Potosi, San Luis Potosi	Nurse, government clinic
Juana[b]	57	Single mother	Tuxpan, Veracruz	Maid, Live-in

[a] The names of the respondents have been changed.
[b] This respondent is coded as a "border-crosser" because she maintains her home in Matamoros, but she lives in Brownsville from Monday through Friday. She works as a live-in maid, but her 16 year-old daughter is allowed to stay with her.

TABLE 2. Characteristics of Women Interviewed in Brownsville

Name	Age	Marital Status	Birthplace	Occupation: United States	Occupation: Mexico
Ninfa	34	Married	Jalpan, Queretaro	Maid for people with disabilities	Farmworker, Maid
Ana	46	Married[a]	Veracruz, Veracruz	Homemaker	Homemaker
Carmen	51	Married	Matamoros, Tamaulipas	Maid	Maid
Norma	40	Married	Matamoros, Tamaulipas	Packer, Shrimp Co.	Farmworker
Alicia	44	Married	Matamoros, Tamaulipas	Farmworker; shrimp packer	Maid, Maquila
Lucia	41	Married	Matamoros, Tamaulipas	None	Maquila
Sonia	35[b]	Widow	Motocintla, Guerrero	Irons clothes, collects cans	None
Letty	35[b]	Single mother	Matamoros, Tamaulipas	Maid	Maid

[a]Husband lives in Mexico
[b]Approximate age

work–good work. They moved to the border because they needed to work but soon became disillusioned at the prospects of meeting their expectations. Because most of the women came with few skills, their marketability was reduced to a very limited status. The life stories of the Matamoros women reflect that work opportunities are sometimes experienced as newfound freedoms. But their life histories also speak to a reality of poor and unfair working conditions and persistent poverty interlaced with these newfound freedoms.

For Lupe, age 24, the lack of opportunity in her hometown highly influenced her decision to migrate north. She explains, "Well, I also came because right now there aren't many work opportunities in the coastal city of Tampico . . . it's rather difficult to find a job there." Lupe's experience reflects how limited employment opportunities for women living in small rural Mexican towns, often motivate their migration to larger urban areas. In Matamoros, job opportunities are concentrated in *maquiladoras*.

Maquiladora work offered both advantages and disadvantages for female workers in that the work provides an immediate source of income, and with time, a few women earned raises and promotions. Gains for the women who migrated in search of work were countered, however, with the common knowledge that companies fired pregnant or older women. Women have a 10 to 15 year time frame for employment in the factories, as Olga explained. "No, right now here if you are 30 years old they will no longer hire you, and they are only hiring the really young women. An older woman thinks twice about leaving her job because she knows that once she quits that she's not going to get another job like this one." Yet, this short working span, the women's earnings provided them a very small income that quite often kept them at the poverty level, and increased the difficulty in their planning for the future.

Lupe was realistic that her impoverished situation remained relatively the same in her new home. It was her perception that her poverty as somewhat alleviated because she was now working and earning her own living. In Lupe's life experience, migration to the border offered her more opportunity because there was access to more jobs. Moreover, at the border the social taboo against women working was less marked. Thus, work provided her a tangible income, and the income gave her a sense of personal independence. Lupe states:

> I believe that the poverty is the same but I do see a difference. There is less work available there [in the interior] and you earn less, so your job provides you less opportunity. I think it's a little bit better here if you spend your money carefully. Moreover, here women can work. Back home the women depend on their husbands to take care of them. So, here if we both work then we can do a bit better.

Upward mobility in the region required more than the subsistence level of income typically earned by these women, and thus these conflicting factors anchored them into a cycle of poverty. A dichotomy of border dynamics existed as catch twenty-two situations for many of the women. Yes, they were now working, a privilege for those coming from small *pueblitos*, rural villages. But the cost of living at the border was much higher than in their hometowns and, in addition, as inexperienced and low-skilled workers, they qualified for the jobs that were least likely to offer upward mobility. While one focus group participant liked her job, she qualified her statement with the meager reality that her income afforded her:

> Where I'm working, I have been there 17 years, and up to now I feel good about working there. The salary isn't very good. A lot of visitors come to our plant and comment on how nice all the women dress at the plant. Yes, they do dress very well, but they also owe a

lot of money just to look good. They must owe a lot because the salaries they pay are not very good. And actually, your pay does not go far enough because everything is so expensive today. If you go out to eat, you'll spend 100 pesos (over $12 U.S.), and for three people [around 300 pesos], and we earn 500 pesos a week ($65 U.S.). From that amount, you have to pay the electricity bill, the water bill and rent.

Women migrate to Mexico's Northern Border with preconceptions and expectations for a better life. The stimulus to the beginning of their internal migration process was based on their life's circumstances in their sending communities. The majority of the women who we interviewed moved to the Border area under arduous circumstances. The process, however, did not change in their new surroundings, as relief in their new home was tempered in coping with the harshness of continued poverty and unfair labor market conditions. Yet, the harshness of their lives was softened when expressed by their personal gains and newfound opportunities. For others, moving to the northern border was one stage in the continuum, and the solution to the improving their life circumstances was to migrate one step further by emigrating across the Border.

EMIGRATION ACROSS THE BORDER INTO THE UNITED STATES

Not surprisingly, the women who settled on the US side of the Border came with new expectations as well, but in many ways their movement across the Border simply reflected an extension of their previous lives in Mexico. The expectation was that migration to the Border would help them find good work, move out of poverty, and build a decent life for their families. Their reasoning seems contradictory given the depressed economy of most US border towns. Nevertheless, for Mexican women living in poverty and with no other options, hope for a better future in the United States sometimes lured them across the Border. The women's life stories revealed their economic insecurity, vulnerability, and fears of apprehension by immigration authorities. While a few women spoke to issues of discrimination, other stories spoke to personal gains and strengths.

Alicia's life history covered her movement across from Matamoros into Brownsville. Her lifestyle and living conditions after she had settled in Brownsville for some time were questioned and criticized by her family who remains in Matamoros. The condition of Alicia's car told her siblings that maybe Alicia was not doing as well as they all had envisioned life in the United States. Alicia explains:

I have family in Matamoros. All of them have their local crossing card and they work in *maquiladoras*, my brothers, my sister and my brother-in-law. I tell them that life is really hard over here [Brownsville]. And they tell me, "Hey, how come you're driving such a rusty car?" . . . And I tell them, "No, it's that working over there [Brownsville] is really difficult and hard." I say, "You have to sweat hard to earn $20 in one day." And then they say, "No, I guess it's better if we stay here [in Matamoros]."

Carmen, on the other hand, felt either country offered her the same options. In Carmen's life story, both places presented obstacles to employment. "I feel it's like being the same. For example, here if you don't have papers, you don't work. Over there [Mexico], if you're not the right age [if you're too old], you don't work. If you don't have an education, well you don't work. So, for me, it's the same [in both countries]." In her opinion a woman with few resources faces many barriers, regardless of whether she lives in the United States or Mexico.

Both women described life in the United States as difficult, and both women appeared disillusioned with their work experiences. Alicia alluded to the fact that it takes more than simply moving to the United States to rise out of poverty. Carmen added that success in the United States requires education and legal immigrant status. A common stereotype among poor Mexicans equates life in the United States with wealth, nice cars and homes, and good jobs. A panoramic view of the United States from the Mexican side of the Border gives the illusion of modernity and prosperity. In Carmen's, Alicia's and the other women's experiences, in spite of high expectations and hard work, life in the United States did not provide the good jobs they moved in search of.

In discussing her precarious situation, Letty, as did many of the other women, explained that her undocumented status placed her and her daughters in an unstable and insecure situation. She pointed to the US employer's willingness to hire poor, undocumented immigrants, like her, to do their worst jobs, experiences that she now recognized as exploitative. Letty's movement across the Border began early in her life with a maid's job in Brownsville, an arrangement made by her parents. It was a job that allowed her to qualify for a day-worker's permit. Letty's words rang with the fears of a young woman and at the same time with the expectations and needs of her family. "I came over here at age 18 [under a day-workers permit] . . . I worked and would send money by telegraph to my parents. This was so they wouldn't have to cross and so that I wouldn't have to cross either. "Right? Because, I was so scared [of crossing back and forth]. And, I didn't know anyone here. No one. Absolutely no one."

Eighteen years later and still living without legal documentation, her words were calloused and critical of the life she had come to experience in the United States. She feels that Mexicans in the United States have not had the opportunity to rise beyond the worse jobs–working in the fields, washing cars, cleaning houses–and she attributes this to racial discrimination. Letty's hardened beliefs reflect a lifetime of limited opportunities.

The jobs that Letty and Alicia held were those of domestic maids, the low-paying jobs that come without benefits or potential for upward mobility. Steady employment was highly valued regardless of whether it fell on the US or the Mexican side of the Border; but given the women's limited resources and Brownsville's high unemployment rate, the women in Brownsville faced a challenge in creating that good life they came searching for. Clearly, the women's undocumented status coupled with their very poor occupational skills inhibited their ability to capitalize on the fact that they lived within a transnational setting.

Ana and her family had known poverty in Mexico, and their life story highlighted how the new life they established in Brownsville offered no luxuries. They settled in one of Brownsville's outlying *colonias*. Home for the family of seven was a room that measured no more than 6' by 9' with an attached kitchen that measured approximately 3' by 4' and an outhouse. Yet, there was a source of pride this immigrant family showed in the brightly painted exterior of their sleeping quarters. Ana was proud too that it was a home with running water and electricity, as these basic services were luxuries where she came from. Ana viewed having these services as an accomplishment in that she and other women had worked hard to gain them in their *colonia*. Thus, the gains represented much more; they exemplified their ability to apply the survival strategies they brought with them to this new environment. Despite the impoverished conditions in which this family of seven lived, this was their own home and they viewed it as an asset they had gained in their lives. Ana detailed their life's experience:

> I still don't know it [the Border area]. I hardly ever go out. Well, it's like in all places because for us, who are here without papers,

we struggle a lot. Before, many of us didn't have water and we had to carry it [at our homes in Mexico]. So, we continue in poverty, but here most of us here have water. We have water and electricity. We went through some very tough times because at first we didn't have water or electricity. And to not have a car [here]. You see that without a car here you're no one. But, thanks to God, it's been 4 years since we first came and we're fine now. We're poor here. My kids haven't gone hungry. They've had food to eat, not a whole lot, but before we came from a ranch where life was very hard.

The women living in Brownsville migrated with the expectation that they would build a better life for themselves. Although they achieved very low levels of economic success, they still saw their homes and life in the United States as a positive accomplishment. Most placed a high significance on working regardless of the work conditions. Again, the opportunity to work was viewed as an achievement and seen as a personal gain toward independence. But many of the women's perceptions of their gains did not necessarily match the harsh reality of their lives, but for all of the women hope lay in their children's futures.

INTEGRATION AND SETTLEMENT AT THE BORDER

Successful integration in both the United States and Mexico were examined on the basis of economic, institutional and interpersonal. Economic integration applies to employment issues, including job accessibility and maintenance. Institutional integration focuses on whether individuals participate in social and public organizations. Social and family interactions make up the interpersonal component (Hondagneu Sotelo, 1994; Marquez, 1998; Massey, 1986).

Work opportunities have increased in Matamoros as in most other large Northern Border towns. Unfortunately, these opportunities primarily related directly to the maquiladoras, an industry that presents more shortterm employment, rather than "good lifetime job opportunities" (Escobar & Roberts, 1998, p. 39). Access to employment opportunities remained a key settlement predictor for poor women at the Mexican Border zone. In their situation, successful settlement included more long term employment, and access to the more stable jobs–the jobs usually reserved for the male employees (Escobar & Roberts, Marquez, 1998; 1998; Pena, 1997). The women's situation in Brownsville was more complex, and, as a result, successful settlement for Brownsville's female, immigrant population required skillful negotiation on all three levels: the economic, interpersonal, and institutional level.

The women in Matamoros achieved a very moderate level of economic success. This moderate level of success was based on the fact that all but one was employed in the formal labor market. The small amount of success achieved had limited affects as they all earned salaries so low that the majority could not support a family on this income. The Brownsville women achieved very low levels of economic success based on their limited access to jobs and reliance on seasonal jobs. The women were either unemployed or worked as domestic maids, ironing clothes, or in low-paying factory jobs. All in all, any gains achieved by the women were negated by their concentration in gender-segregated jobs and/or gender typed jobs, very long workdays, and poor working conditions.

Regarding institutional integration, the Brownsville women gained limited access to social and public organizations. The lack of legal documentation was highly significant in keeping the women away from public and social organizations. Another contributing factor was the women were forced to settle in marginalized *colonia* communities. Other barriers included low levels of education, limited English language skills, and lack of transportation. Meaningful success in terms of institutional integration, however, did occur in that their children attended local public schools. One could argue that this success must be qualified in that their schools were close to their *colonia*, and *colonias* are marginalized communities in their own right. The residents of Cameron Park would argue otherwise, as they worked hard to gain an elementary school within the perimeter of their colonia. Thus, the school's presence is viewed as a community asset.

The women in Matamoros achieved a moderate level of social and public integration aided by the fact that illegal immigrant status was not a factor with which to contend with. The women expressed the positive gains of remaining in Mexico: the freedom to move about; voting rights; and access to public institutions such as the Mexican social security system. Nevertheless, the majority of the women were still hampered by their limited education, and extremely long working hours. The former reduced the women's ability to raise their social status, and the latter limited their interactions with others outside of their work environment. Moreover, the women's inadequate incomes made it difficult for them to help their children obtain a better education within the current structure of the Mexican public school system.

In Brownsville, the women achieved little success in terms of interpersonal integration in the form of social interactions and family interactions outside of the *colonia* where they lived. They often remained marginalized from the broader Brownsville community as a result of a paralyzing fear of apprehension by the Border Patrol, long work days that left no time for outside activities, and their time consuming and burdensome role as primary caretakers of the family. Outside friendships and contacts were extremely limited and new friendships were mostly confined to their *colonia*. In fact, the women's existence was basically confined to the *colonia*, except for those who worked in town. Some women, however, were active participants in their colonia's community center, taking English classes, immigration regulations and procedure classes, health care instruction and many additional life-skill classes. One highly significant gain that many of the Brownsville women achieved was in their movement towards personal independence compared to what they had experienced in Mexico. Key to this point is that the Brownsville women were older and from a different generation, and they expressed their personal success and gains by their contributions in the decision making process required of them by the settlement process. Prior to immigration, their husbands tended to make all the decisions.

The women in Matamoros, too, experienced a significant level of success in their achievement of interpersonal integration but at a higher level and for different reasons. They were not confined to the *colonia* in which they lived, and had freedom of movement throughout the town. Equally important, the majority of the women had a strong family network (as most upon arrival were received by a relative), and drew from a solid family support network eventually expanding outwards with new friendships.

IMPLICATIONS FOR SOCIAL SERVICE PROVISION TO IMMIGRANTS ON THE US-MEXICAN BORDER

Clearly, transnational forces in the US-Mexico region uniquely express themselves in the migration histories of the women who live there. We presented information gathered from migration life histories of women in poverty living in this region, one group who had migrated from the interior of Mexico to the northern Mexican border and a second group who had immigrated across the border to the United States. We found that the migration experience of women is often characterized by poverty and very poor living conditions, particularly among those residing in *colonias*. At the same time, they have demonstrated that their survival strategies are creative and adaptive, and they have been successful in improving the living conditions within their *colonias*. For many, arrival at the Border reflected only a stage in migration, before continuing on to the United States in search of better economic opportunities. A key finding in this study was that women in poverty who migrate to the Border area face limited success in terms of economic, institutional, and personal integration. Thus, the life histories present evidence that the transnational elements involved in migration to the Texas-Mexico Borderlands further adds to an already complex, uprooting process.

The knowledge gained from this study provides a better understanding of the needs of immigrants living on the US northern border with Mexico and a guide to the design of effective social service provision. Three specific approaches include promoting bi-national collaborative efforts, helping immigrants living in *colonias* improve their communities, and designing programs that help very low-income immigrants move toward full integration:

* Binational collaborative efforts for social service provision are imperative in this region due to its transnational character. Bi-national programs in health services, such as the *United States-Mexico Border Health Association*, provide a model for social service collaboration.
* The *US-Mexico Border Health Association* promotes health along the US-Mexico border through reciprocal technical cooperation, dissemination of information and the creation of networks. It also supports sister city relationships through its Binational Health Councils and facilitates partnership building among the public and private sectors.
* Provision of services to immigrants living in *colonias* requires helping residents to organize for the creation and/or facilitation of access to services. For example, *The Colonias Program* is designed to assist *colonia* residents to strengthen the social infrastructure of the community (*Colonias* Program, n.d.). The program works in partnership with local government, state and federal agencies, nonprofit organizations, and promotes the active involvement of residents. The program helps *colonia* residents access education, health and human services, job training, youth and elderly programs available in their areas.
* In order to assist very low-income immigrants on the border to fully integrate into US society, several specific barriers need to be addressed: legal status, low education and job skills, and poor access to public and social institutions. Services may include citizenship programs, classes in English as a Second Language, and outreach geared specifically to this population (Padilla, 1997).

PROSPECTS OF IMMIGRATION POLICY
FOR THE US-MEXICO BORDER

Overall, Mexican immigration to the United States has significant and complicated implications for policy. Under the current presidential administrations, Mexico and the United States began discussions to readdress the issue of Mexican immigration. In a joint statement between the United States and Mexico made on September 6, 2001, the Presidents from both countries "renewed their commitment to forging new and realistic approaches to migrations" (White House, 2001). Both Presidents agreed this includes the process of "matching willing workers with willing employers" (White House, 2001). Furthermore, they agreed future immigration discussion must focus on "respecting the human dignity of all migrants, regardless of status; recognizing the contribution migrants make to enriching both societies; shared responsibility for ensuring migration takes place through safe and legal channels" (Joint Statement, 2001).

Although possibilities for immigration reform were received with great anticipation, the terrorist attacks against the United States that occurred on September 11, 2001, placed immigration policy on the backburner. Homeland security has become a national priority and has resulted in increased efforts aimed at tightening the US borders. With the tightening of the borders, entry into the United States has become more difficult. The negative impact on the economy, which has resulted in reduced jobs, has also resulted in decreased immigration. Furthermore, it is estimated that more than 350,000 Mexicans have returned to Mexico because they've lost their jobs (Sullivan & Jordan, 2001a; Dillon, 2001). For now, discussions on a "bilateral agenda" have stalled, although there is some agreement among legislators that talks will begin anew at the beginning of 2002 and that Congress will pass immigration reform legislation later in the year (Sullivan & Jordan, 2001, November 18, 2001; November 15).

SUGGESTED READINGS AND SOURCES OF INFORMATION

Center for Immigration Research: *http://www.uh.edu/cir/*
Center for Comparative Immigration Studies, University of California-San Diego. *www.ccis-ucsd.org*
Colonias *www.sos.state.tx.us/border/colonias/*
Hondagneu-Sotelo, P. (2001). *Doméstica: Immigrant workers cleaning and caring in the shadows of affluence.* Berkeley: University of California Press.
Oropesa, R. S. & Landale, N. S. (1997). Immigrant legacies: ethnicity, generation, and children's familial and economic lives. *Social Science Quarterly*, 78(2), 399-416.

Rumbaut, R. G. & Portes, A. (2001). *Ethnicities: children of immigrants in America.* New York: Russell Sage Foundation.
TEXAS COLONIA PROJECT . www.twdb.state.tx.us/colonias/
Trueba, E. T. (1999). *Latinos unidos: From cultural diversity to the politics of solidarity.* Lanham, MA: Rowman & Littlefield.

REFERENCES

Baca-Zinn, M. (1998). Hispanic American families in the United States: Adaptation and continuity in Mexican-origin families. In Taylor, R. (Ed.), *Minority families in the United States: A multicultural perspective* (pp. 77-94), NJ: Prentice Hall.

Bean F., de la Garza, R., Roberts, B., & Weintraub S. (Eds.). (1997). *At the crossroads: Mexico and U.S. immigration policy.* Lanham, MD: Rowman & Littlefield, Publishers, Inc.

Colonias factbook. (1988). Texas Department of Human Services. Austin, Texas.

Colonias program. (n.d.). Center for housing and urban development. Texas A & M University: Bryan, Texas. Retrieved October 25, 2002, from http://chud.tamu.edu/

Colonias program: *Colonias* in Texas. (2000). Center for housing and urban development. Texas A & M University: Bryan, Texas.

Curry-Rodriguez, J. (1988). Labor migration and familial responsibilities: Experiences of Mexican women. *Mexicanas at work in the United States.* Houston, TX: University of Texas, Mexican American studies program.

Dillon, S. (2001, Oct. 15), Mexican immigrants face new set of fears. *New York Times.* New York, NY, p. 14A.

Drachman, D. (1992). A stage-of-migration framework for service to immigrant populations. *Social Work,* 37, 68-72.

Escobar-Lapati, A. & Roberts, B. (1998). Migration and economic development along the U.S.- Mexico border. Austin, TX: Population Research Center.

Gelbard, A. & Carter, M. (1997). Mexican immigration and the U.S. population. In Bean, F. et al. (Ed.), *At the crossroads: Mexico and United States immigration policy* (pp. 117-144). Lanham, MD: Rowman & Littlefield, Publishers, Inc.

Gonzalez, S., Ruiz, O., Velasco, L. & Woo, O. (Compiladoras). (1995). *Mujeres, migracion y maquila en la frontera norte. El Colegio de la Frontera Norte, El Colegio de Mexico: Mexico, D.F.*

Hondagneu-Sotelo, P. (1994). *Gendered transitions: Mexican experiences of immigration.* Berkeley, CA: University of California Press.

Lein, L. & Padilla, Y. (1997). Hispanic children on the Texas-Mexican border. *Perspectivas Sociales/Social Perspectives,* 1(1), 77-86.

Maril, R. (1989). *Poorest of Americans: The Mexican-Americans of the Lower Rio Grande Valley of Texas.* Notre Dame, Indiana: University of Notre Dame Press.

Marquez, R. (1998). *Migration processes: Impoverished women immigrants along the Texas/Mexico border.* Unpublished doctoral dissertation, The University of Texas at Austin, Austin, Texas.

Marrujo, O. R. y Ortiz L. V. (1995). *Mujeres en la frontera norte: Su presencia en la migracion y la industria maquiladora. En* Gonzalez, S., Ruiz O., Velasco L. y Woo,

O. (Compiladoras) *Mujeres, Migracion y Maquila en la Frontera Norte.* (pp. 13-36). Tijuana, BC: El Colegio de la Frontera Norte.

Massey, D. (1986). The settlement process among Mexican migrants to the United States. *American Sociological Review, 51*: 670-85.

Padilla, Y. (1997). Immigrant policy: Issues for social work practice. *Social Work, 42* (6), 595- 606.

Padilla, Y., & Daigle, L. (1996). Social and economic interdependence in the United States- Mexico border region: Critical implications for social welfare. *New Global Development: Journal of International and Comparative Social Welfare, 12,* 65-77.

Padilla, Y., Lein, L., & Cruz, M. (1999). Community-based research in policy planning: A case study–addressing poverty in the United States-Mexico border region. *Journal of Community Practice, 6* (4), 1-22.

Peña, D. (1997). *The terror of the machine: Technology, work, gender, and ecology on the United States-Mexico border.* Austin, Texas: CMAS Books, The University of Texas at Austin.

Portes, A. & Bach, R. (1985). *Latin journey: Cuban and Mexican immigrants in the United States.* Berkeley, CA: University of California Press.

Reviere, R., Berkowitz S., Carter, C., & Ferguson, C. (1996). *Needs assessment: A creative and practical guide for social scientists.* Philadelphia, PA: Taylor & Francis.

Roberts, B. & Escobar-Lapati, A. (1997). Mexican social and economic policy and emigration. In Bean, F. et al. (Ed.), *At the crossroads: Mexico and United States immigration policy* (pp. 47- 78). Lanham, MD: Rowman & Littlefield, Publishers, Inc.

Schmidley, A. & Gibson, C. (1999). *Profile of the foreign-born population in the United States: 1997.* Washington, DC: United States Census Bureau, United States Government Printing Office. (Current Population Reports, Series P23-195). Available: http://www.census.gov/prod/99pubs/p23-195.pdf

Strauss, A. & Corbin, J. (1990). Acculturation, access to care, and use of preventive services by Hispanics: Findings from HANES 1982-84. *American Journal of Public Health, 80* (11-19).

Sullivan, K. & Jordan, M. (2001a, November, 18). Daschle, Gephardt visit Mexico. *Washington Post,* p. 34A.

Sullivan, K. & Jordan, M. (2001b, November, 15). United States and Mexico to resume talks on immigration policy; Issue will be recast as one of national security; Daschel, Gephardt to meet with Vicente Fox. *Washington Post,* p. 40A.

Texas comptroller of public accounts. (1998). *Bordering the future: Challenge and opportunity in the Texas border region.* Austin, Texas.

U.S.-Mexico Border Health Association. (n.d.). Retrieved October 25, 2002, from http://www.usmbha.org

Ward, P. (1999). *Colonias and public policy in Texas and Mexico: Urbanization by stealth.* Austin, Texas: University of Texas Press.

Watson, L. & Watson-Franke, M. (1985). *Interpreting Life Histories.* New Brunswick, New Jersey: Rutgers University Press.

Whitehouse. (2001, September 6). An official text of the: "Joint statement between the United States of America and the United Mexican States." Office of the press secretary: Washington, DC. Whitehouse.gov.

Zavella, P. (1993). Feminist insider dilemmas: Constructing ethnic identity with Chicana informants. *A Journal of Women Studies, 13*(3), 138-159.

APPENDIX.

Teaching Point:

Colonias along the Texas-Mexico border

Colonias are rural, unincorporated residential areas that were developed along the US/Mexico border in part as a response to the housing needs of poor Mexican immigrant families. Today, however, the majority of *colonia* residents are US-born. As a result of lack of state regulations, as many as 1450 *colonias* have developed in Texas. Most came into being around the 1970s, although a few–as in the El Paso area–have existed for several centuries. Most *colonias* lack basic commodities, including paved streets, electricity, accessible and clean water, indoor plumbing and sewage disposal systems, and local fire and police protection (*Colonias* program, 2000; *Colonia* factbook, 1988; Ward, 1999). Residents of *colonias* have very high levels of poverty and low educational and occupational levels.

The Lower Rio Grande Valley's 435 *colonias*, where our US respondents lived, comprise close to one-third of all the *colonias* within Texas. Although *colonias* have more recently received attention from legislators and state agencies, they remain pockets of concentrated poverty that are frequently geographically, socially, and legally isolated.

Armenian Refugees
and Displaced Persons
and the Birth of Armenian Social Work

Nancy A. Humphreys

Ludmila Haroutunian

SUMMARY. This article explores the historical and recent patterns of Armenian emigration and immigration and the impact that the population shifts have had and are having. The interconnections between peoples' homeland and new land and the intersection among institutions in the homeland and new land are illustrated. The development of social work as a profession along with a variety of non-governmental organizations in Armenia developed through a unique collaboration between a school of social work in the United States and the major university in Armenia is discussed and illustrated. *[Article copies available for a fee from The Haworth Document Delivery Service: 1-800-HAWORTH. E-mail address: <docdelivery@haworthpress.com> Website: <http://www.HaworthPress.com> © 2004 by The Haworth Press, Inc. All rights reserved.]*

Nancy A. Humphreys, DSW, ACSW, is Professor and Director, Institute for the Advancement of Political Social Work Practice, University of Connecticut School of Social Work.

Ludmila Haroutunian is Chair, Department of Sociology, Social Work and Conflictology, Yerevan State University, Republic of Armenia.

[Haworth co-indexing entry note]: "Armenian Refugees and Displaced Persons and the Birth of Armenian Social Work." Humphreys, Nancy A., and Ludmila Haroutunian. Co-published simultaneously in *Journal of Immigrant & Refugee Services* (The Haworth Social Work Practice Press, an imprint of The Haworth Press, Inc.) Vol. 2, No. 1/2, 2004, pp. 31-48; and: *Immigrants and Social Work: Thinking Beyond the Borders of the United States* (ed: Diane Drachman, and Ana Paulino) The Haworth Social Work Practice Press, an imprint of The Haworth Press, Inc., 2004, pp. 31-48. Single or multiple copies of this article are available for a fee from The Haworth Document Delivery Service [1-800-HAWORTH, 9:00 a.m. - 5:00 p.m. (EST). E-mail address: docdelivery@haworthpress.com].

KEYWORDS. Armenia, Armenian diaspora, refugees, displaced persons, nongovernmental organizations, Armenian social work

INTRODUCTION

The Armenian people have been defined, both in ancient and modern times, by complex patterns of migration. At the beginning of the 21st Century it is estimated that there are six million Armenians world-wide. The first official census since Armenia became an independent republic was conducted in October of 2000. However, complete results and analysis are not expected until late 2003 (Gareginian, 11/2001 *AIM*). The last official counting of the population, while the country was still a part of the Soviet Union in 1989, put the country's population at more than three million residents. The accuracy of this number is suspect, given the disorganization and lack of resources associated with the final days of the Soviet Union. In addition, a large number of Armenians live outside the country. Approximately half of all Armenians live in the world wide diaspora . A large number of Armenians live in France, Syria, Iran, Israel and other countries in the Middle East. Approximately one million Armenians live in the United States. The Armenians living in the diaspora have and continue to play an important role in the maintenance of Armenia and Armenian culture. The story of migration to and from Armenia includes a fierce loyalty that most Armenians share in their collective ethnic history and culture.

The purpose of this article is to explore historical and recent patterns of Armenian emigration and immigration. Discussion includes the significant impact these population shifts have had and are having on the culture, the people, and the country of Armenia. The emergence of social work and a school of social work in Armenia that derives in part from the contributions of Armenian immigrants in the diaspora is described. The presentation also illustrates the interconnection between people's homeland and new land and the interaction among institutions in the homeland and new land that emerges out of migration.

The territory now occupied by Armenia has been at the cross road, and sometimes the actual battlefield, of many political and religious struggles throughout history continuing to current times. As a result, the country's political borders have changed many times while the culture and ethnic identity have remained stable surviving both conquest and official efforts to diminish the Armenian culture or eliminate Armenians as a distinct people. The repeated political struggles over territory lead to large numbers of Armenian being displaced and complex patterns of migration.

Armenia today is a newly independent small landlocked Christian country in the southern Caucasus region. It became a free and independent country in 1991 with the break up of the Soviet Union. The newly independent and free republic represents only the most recent representation of Armenia. Armenians trace their unique culture, if not discrete territory, to the 6th century B.C. It is the oldest continuous Christian country in the world. The advent of the 21st century marks the 1700th anniversary of the Armenian Christian Church which has survived and served as the keeper of the Armenian culture and language even during Soviet times, when the celebration of religion and separate ethnic and culture identities were officially forbidden.

Armenian migration patterns have been and continue to be complex. The first large scale genocide of the 20th century began with the massacre and displacement of more than a million and a half Armenians in a land grab by the Ottoman Empire from an area, then known as Western Armenia. While the world stood by, largely silent, more than a million and a half Armenians were forced to flee their homes, perhaps as many as a million were murdered. The massacre and removal of Armenians represents the first of the major attempts at the genocide of a people that has defined the 20th century. During World War II when the Third Reich was contemplating the "final solution" of the "Jewish question," Hitler, when asked if he thought the world would tolerate such systematic genocide, asked, "Who remembers the Armenians?" While no specific source has been found for this remark, it is widely repeated. Some argue that it might be apocryphal (Balakian, 1997). This effort to displace ethnic Armenians from territory they had lived on for centuries was the first example of what would later come to be known as "ethnic cleansing."

ARMENIAN DIASPORA

The Armenians who fled the genocide formed the first generation of refugees in the diaspora which has played a continuing and important role in the life of Armenia and the Armenian people. Many of those who fled became well established and assimilated in their new countries. However, they never lost, at least not completely, their attachment to and identification with the Armenian territory as well as its rich and long cultural traditions. In some cases this identity may have been little more than the continuation of distinct surnames, the familiar "ian" which became a symbol of Armenian ethnicity in English speaking countries. Despite the repeated efforts, by many different groups and governments, to annihilate or force their assimilation, Armenians have, in the main, remained a clearly identified ethnic group with their own culture. This has been equally true for those in the geographic homeland as well as those in the world-wide diaspora. The world famous poet and Armenian folk hero William Saroyan portrays Armenian ethnic identity as he writes:

> I should like to see any power in this world destroy this race, this small tribe of unimportant people whose history is ended, whose wars have been fought and lost, whose structures have crumbled, whose literature is unread, whose music is unheard and whose prayers are no more answered. Go ahead, destroy this! Destroy Armenia! See if you can do it. Send them from their homes into the desert. Let them have neither bread nor water. Burn their homes and churches. Then see if they will not laugh again, see if they will not sing and pray again. For when two of them meet anywhere in the world, see if they will not create a New Armenia. (Quoted in Elektron)

Nowhere were the efforts to extinguish the Armenian culture more prevalent than in the policies of the former Soviet Union which subjected separate cultural and ethnic identities to rigid central authority. One of the official policies of the Soviet Union, particularly harshly imposed during the reign of Joseph Stalin, resulted in the wholesale uprooting and relocation of members of one ethnic group into the territory of another. The official purpose of this policy was to make ethnic identity hard to maintain and allegiance to central authority more likely. As a result of this policy many Armenians were forcibly resettled to other regions throughout the Soviet Union. A large number of Armenians were relocated to neighboring Azerbaijan, a Muslim country with longstanding ethnic hostilities toward their Christian Armenian neighbors. The relocated Armenians were settled in a territory which came to be known as Nagorno Karabakh.

POST SOVIET ERA

During the time of the break up of the Soviet Union, the ethnic Armenians in the Karabakh demanded the right to become an independent country or as an alternative to become a part of Armenia. The government of Azerbaijan refused and war erupted between the Karabakh and Azerbaijan. Later the hostilities were actively supported by the newly independent Republic of Armenia. After years of intense fighting and escalating hostilities, a cease fire was agreed to in 1994. The future of this disputed territory, as well as sizeable areas of Azerbaijan which came under Armenian occupation and control during the war, await final settlement.

The war and its aftermath affected Armenia (and Azerbaijan) in many ways. During the period of hostilities large numbers of residents on both sides of the border were unable to remain in their homes due to frequent and persistent shelling. Many residents fled their homes and moved to safer more protected areas of their respective countries. Some of the Armenians chose to leave the Karabakh and became residents in Armenian territory, a population shift fully sanctioned by the newly formed national government in Armenia. During the years when the war was most intense, Armenia was subjected to a total blockade of its borders with the technical exception of Georgia to the north. Turkey and Iran, both Muslim countries and strong supporters of Azerbaijan, refused to allow any people or goods to move through its borders. Even the airspace was forbidden to Armenian air traffic. While the border with Georgia remained open most of the time and air traffic was permitted through its airspace, it was beset by its own internal civil war which made the border dangerous and the movement of goods and services unpredictable. In the early years of the Republic, the only outside source of energy was a gas line that ran through Georgia. The line was cut or sabotaged as often as it was in operation. During these years, Armenia suffered severe energy shortages and draconian rationing which made everyday life extremely difficult.

Armenians throughout the diaspora, most especially Armenian-Americans, were instrumental in helping the new country through contributions of humanitarian assistance and putting political pressure to force neighboring governments, especially Turkey who has strong ties to the West to open its borders and enable goods and services to move into Armenia. Lifting the blockade, which happened in 1995, required the intervention of and leverage by the United States using the threat of the loss of foreign aid to Turkey unless the blockade was lifted (H.R. 1868, 1995).

Another very difficult cost of the conflict was the forced expulsion or decision to flee made by ethnic Armenians who lived in Azerbaijan, not the Karabakh. Likewise, large numbers of ethnic Azerbaijanis were expelled or fled Armenia. In addition, Armenians living in other newly independent countries of the former Soviet Union fearing ethnic-political conflicts also fled to Armenia. These fears were particularly keen for those Armenians who lived in countries where Islam was to become the dominant religion or where Muslims were the majority ethnic group. The fear of being persecuted played a significant role in the migration patterns among all of the newly independent states. Most of those who fled the Karabakh, Azerbaijan or other former Soviet countries were pushed from their homes and countries in which they were citizens. Like most refugees who are forced to leave they did so with great reservations. According to State proclamations by the former Soviet Union, principles of shared political citizenship and an integrated civil society, which respected the rights of all citizens equally were promoted. However, almost all post-Soviet countries have been dominated by conflict between and among ethnic groups with minority groups feeling vulnerable. The seventy year plus efforts of the USSR to reduce ethnic identification and create ethnically neutral social and political relationships failed. Today most of the newly formed states are organized along ethnic lines or religious preferences.

    In some instances the old ethnic tensions have broken out into war. Currently, the world community pays large sums of money to forcibly keep peace among groups that would otherwise be at war.

    Between 1988 and 1992, 360,000 refugees arrived in Armenia from Azerbaijan and Nagorno Karabakh. These people were refugees in every sense of the United Nations definition. They were forced to leave because of persecution. They were unable to remain or return to their native country and they sought the protection of the state to which they fled (Van Wormer 1997). The most significant difference between these refugees and others was that the vast majority of them were ethnic Armenians who had never lived or visited the country. The newly independent republic lacked resources to meet the needs of the new arrivals as well as those of its own citizens. In addition, the "State" was unable to provide sufficient economic opportunities for people to work and earn a living because of the quick change from the Soviet economic system that guaranteed jobs for all to a system based on free market principles where individuals and families are responsible for themselves. The change in government and in the economic system associated with the break-up of the Soviet Union resulted in major social and economic problems. Unemployment, underemployment, rampant poverty and a dramatic increase in crime and corruption occurred. As Midgely (1997) notes the collapse of Communism brought serious reversals in the quality of life for ordinary citizens.

During the arrival of the greatest number of refugees, Armenia experienced a devastating earthquake in heavily populated areas of the northeastern part of the country. Twenty-five thousand persons died and more than 300,000 were left homeless and without work. Promises were made by the central government in Moscow that economic relief and new housing would be provided. However, aid did not materialize due to lack of resources. Local government also had few resources to address the overwhelming need. As a result, local Armenian authorities and the Soviet government took the unprecedented step of making it easier for outsiders, especially Armenians from the diaspora, to come to Armenia and help with relief efforts. Hundreds, perhaps thousands, of Armenians from the diaspora came to Armenia to help with the aftermath of the effects of the earthquake. For many, this marked their first time visiting Armenia. Despite never having been there, the nation and the people of Armenia had been kept alive through the stories and the struggles told to them by their parents and grandparents. Many of the ethnic Armenians in the diaspora contributed concrete assistance and material aid to extended family and strangers. Large amounts of economic aid and humanitarian relief, much of it from Armenian Americans flowed into the country as a result of the government's new openness to outside help and relaxed trade and travel restrictions.

The Armenians from the diaspora have become a critical economic resource to the new Republic. Large sums of humanitarian aid now regularly flow into the country and many Armenians in the diaspora regularly send money to relatives, often family they have never met given the rigidity of the earlier Soviet travel restrictions. Voluntary assistance from extended family members in the diaspora makes up a significant proportion of family income and a significant part of the country's gross domestic product. The Armenian Assembly of America, a major organization that represents the interests of Armenia and Armenians living in the United States, places the current gross domestic product (GDP) of Armenia at 2.1 billion dollars of which 300 million dollars come from the diaspora. This means that almost one sixth of the Armenian (GDP) comes from the descendants of refugees throughout the diaspora. In addition Armenians who send money to family also commonly participate in family decision making. Similarly, those who contribute humanitarian assistance to the country as a whole believe that they have a right and an obligation to pay attention and in some instances seek to influence the internal social, political and economic system in the country.

THE NEW REPUBLIC
AND THE INCREASE OF DISPLACED PERSONS

The serendipitous intersection of three cataclysmic events, the earthquake, the break up of the Soviet Union and a significant influx of refugees dominated the early years of the new Republic. These events resulted in significant deprivation among a sizeable population, considerable distrust of government, and social strife. Nowhere was this collision of social forces more clear than in the escalating housing crisis. The arrival of refugees and persons displaced by the earthquake made an already critical housing shortage much worse. Refugees and earthquake victims shared a similar status as internally displaced persons who lacked basic resources and few opportunities to remedy their deprivation (Van Wormer, 1997). Their situation was made worse by the inability of the government to plan for or meet the needs of internally displaced individuals and families. The new Armenian government could not meet the need for housing and outside humanitarian assistance could not keep pace with the escalating need for shelter. The needs of earthquake survivors and the refugee population were similar despite the fact that the origin of their situation was different.

Because of the similarities between refugees and other groups of displaced persons, Ahearn (1995) argues that both groups could be included in a single category of displaced persons. Both are forced to flee their homes and both groups are without basic resources. In contrast, Alaverdyan (2001) argues for a more finite categorization of displaced persons. In respect to modern day Armenia, she divides displaced persons into broad categories based on where they came from: (Azerbaijan, a border area, other former Soviet territory, or the diaspora); and how they came to Armenia (were they deported, did they flee, were they forced out, or did they leave voluntarily)? When using specific categorization, it is necessary to place many persons in more than one category.

The finite categorization of displaced persons facilitates differentiation among the circumstances of refugees or immigrants and earthquake survivors. The differentiation makes it possible to argue for compensation that would be appropriate for different groups of displaced persons. For example, many Armenians including many in the government, argue that significant compensation should be forthcoming from the government of Azerbaijan who, they claim is responsible for the dislocation of many of those who fled Azerbaijan. (Not surprising the government of Azerbaijan argues that Armenia should be responsible for paying for the cost of those who fled from Armenia to Azerbaijan.) Distinguishing those refugees who came from Azerbaijan from others who migrated to Armenia would be necessary in order to sustain the argument of governmental responsibility. The issue of reparations for those who lost their homes and possessions as a result of the war and official governmental policies and actions remains to be settled in a final solution of the war between Armenian and Azerbaijan.

Activities associated with the movement of refugees, earthquake survivors and other displaced persons and the governments responses can be grouped into three distinct phases. During the first phase, the period between 1988 and 1991, large numbers of refugees from Azerbaijan were forced to flee to Armenia (and vice versa) in response to the war. Many residents in villages on the Armenian side of the border were also forced to flee to safer locations in response to the persistent shelling. During the same time the earthquake added hundreds of thousands of survivors who were displaced from their homes and jobs as whole communities were left with no livable space and no economic infrastructure or activity.

Between 1992 and 1995, the middle phase in the movement of refugees and displaced persons, large numbers of refugees continued to arrive from Azerbaijan. At the same time a new group of refugees, specifically Armenians who had been living in other areas of the Soviet Union, returned to Armenia out of fear for their safety. Many of the newly independent republics in the former Soviet Union were strong supporters of Azerbaijan and the ethnic Armenians who lived there feared that they might not be protected by the new governments. The government of Armenia welcomed Armenians to their cultural home as a symbol of the viability of the newly independent country. This policy also encouraged the migration of Armenians who had never lived in Armenia. They were returning to a shared culture and ethnic identification as a protection against common enemies both geographic and cultural. During this phase, there was also outmigration. Some Armenians left the country because they were afraid of their fate in the newly free country. These Armenians had been supportive of the Soviet system and resisted independence. Other native Armenians took advantage of fairly open immigration policies in countries with large Armenian populations. They left because they viewed the social and political transition would be difficult. Some joined family who had immigrated to other countries in years past.

In 1995, the Law of Citizenship was passed. The law granted refugees the right to become citizens of Armenia. This marked the beginning of the third and current phase of refugee migration patterns into and out of Armenia. The number of refugees from Azerbaijan and other republics of the former Soviet Union decreased. However, the majority of those who had arrived earlier remained in temporary overcrowded housing and in congested communities. Some lived in refugee settlements with access to few social or economic resources. Likewise, the majority of earthquake survivors continued to live in temporary arrangements. Their previous social experience with the government which provided for their basic needs led them to wait for an institution to improve their situation. Further outmigration also occurred during this phase. Thousands of skilled Armenians left to work in other countries, especially Russia where economic opportunity was greater.

Throughout the three phases of migration activity, the refugees faced problems in becoming integrated into the social order. The vast majority of ethnic Armenians who fled Azerbaijan and other former Soviet republics came to Armenia for the first time. Many did not speak Armenian which had become the official language at the time of independence. Since Russian was the language of instruction in all levels of schools throughout the former Soviet Union, communication was possible among the educated classes. However, as part of their new national identity, speaking Russian was discouraged causing the new arrivals to experience many problems which made them feel out of place. They arrived suspicious of authority and sometimes with the expectation that they should receive preferential treatment from their new country because their suffering came as a result of their ethnicity. In most respects, they were foreigners despite their shared ethnic and cultural identities. In addition, most of those who fled to Armenia came with little more than what they could carry as many had been displaced by armed soldiers. The extent of their deprivation was great and post traumatic stress disorder and related trauma reactions were common among the new arrivals.

In the early years of migration the usual stresses experienced by refugees were made worse by attempts on the part of the central Soviet government to minimize the refugee problem and hide the refugees in order to foster a belief in the outside world that social life was proceeding normally and peacefully during the period of transition. Thus many of the refugees were hidden in government subsidized holiday hotels, vacation houses, or other locations suitable to congregate housing such as temporary encampments or abandoned military or sports training facilities. These locations were in isolated areas away from population centers and void of economic opportunity.

THE DEVELOPMENT
OF SOCIAL WORK AND THE CREATION
OF NON-GOVERNMENTAL ORGANIZATIONS (NGOS)

The newly formed Armenian government lacked the money to support anything other than basic survival services for needy and displaced persons and earthquake survivors. In response to the many problems that plagued the new country, resources poured in from the outside world, especially from the world wide diaspora. The outside resources were more than matched, at least in effort, by ordinary Armenians who helped family members, neighbors and strangers alike and created new and completely novel mutual aid activities. Another important resource was the arrival of experts, again with many coming from the diaspora, who provided professional expertise. The arrival of experts in social work, mental health and other helping professions along with the collaborative activities with persons and institutions in Armenia were instrumental in the birth of social work and the creation of a flourishing community of non-governmental organizations (NGOs).

One collaboration resulted in the development of a school of social work in Armenia. The collaboration was arranged by an American social worker, a son of refugees who fled the Armenian genocide. He spent a year in Armenia after the earthquake developing mental health services for children in the earthquake zone. On a home visit to the United States (U.S.) in 1990 he contacted the University of Connecticut School of Social Work to propose a joint effort to develop western style social work in Armenia. This collaboration was facilitated by a number of factors, including a new program emphasis on international collaboration at the University of Connecticut (UConn) and a general understanding of social work among Yerevan State University (YSU) sociology faculty. The early phases of the newly formed collaboration were assisted by the fact that the head of the YSU Sociology Department had a diplomatic passport, as a member of the Supreme Soviet, which enabled easy travel. The Armenian-American social worker arranged financial support for travel back and forth between the United States and Armenia from a Swiss Foundation that supported work in the country. Central to the success of this collaboration was very strong personal chemistry between the principle collaborators from the very beginning.

A collaboration with a U.S. school of social work was deemed essential by the Armenians as they understood that the social work profession would be needed as Armenia moved from a centralized command and control economic system to a free market economy. The collaboration between the two universities has been aided by the involvement of several projects supported by the European Union and led by the London School of Economics.

The collaboration has taken many forms. One important early activity was UConn's facilitation of a study tour for the head of the YSU sociology faculty where she was able to visit both public and private agency social service programs while also meeting and consulting with a number of UConn faculty on the development of social work education programs in Armenia. A similar study tour of social service agencies and programs was later arranged for the then Minister of Labor and Social Welfare in the first independently elected government in the new Republic of Armenia. Throughout the collaboration there have been frequent visits and consultations among faculty from both universities.

Many educational resources and materials have been sent to Armenia with the help of a prominent and wealthy member of the Armenian diaspora in the United States who pays for shipping a variety of materials to the country. To date more than 30,000 books and journals have been sent to Armenia. These materials have enabled faculty to create a separate specialized social work library for students and faculty. These materials were useful since the faculty and many of the students became English-reading. They were gathered from retiring social work practitioners and faculty in the United States. Through these donations complete collections of the major U.S. professional social work journals, texts and books have been made available. As the program expanded and educational sites were developed in other parts of the country libraries in these places have also received a number of books and publications. Films, videos and audio tapes and the equipment to play them have been sent along with study guides to aid in the training and educating of social workers in Armenia.

The YSU faculty moved quickly to develop social work education and training programs in order to get as many people as possible prepared to help people who were caught up in the dramatic economic transition that followed independence from the former Soviet Union. The first programs involved a series of six month training programs intended to give those trained enough knowledge and beginning skills to enable them to help individual, groups and communities and develop programs to cope with the high rates of unemployment, underemployment and poverty that immediately followed the conversion to a free market economy. These short term training programs were tailored for government and NGO employees and others who were to become the first generation of trained social service workers in Armenia. The training concentrated on helping techniques and emphasized a combination of classroom instruction with field work training.

Following the completion and evaluation of the training programs the YSU faculty introduced a five year undergraduate degree in social work to be pursued by sociology majors. Eventually the department of sociology was re-named to include social work and social work became a separate major. Shortly after the implementation of the new social work program the university as a whole, following the pattern typical in the West, decided to move from five year to four year undergraduate degree programs. After graduating two cohorts of undergraduate social work majors, the faculty with encouragement of YSU administrators created a one year Masters in Social Work Program. The program was open to graduates of the undergraduate program only. Thus a total of five years consisting of undergraduate and graduate programs became the highest level of social work training available. UConn faculty and staff offered consultations on course development and curriculum organization and gathered teaching and learning resources to augment didactic teaching.

The "Social Work" faculty were in reality trained sociologists, most of whom had PhDs, but had no actual social work experience. Throughout the collaboration, UConn faculty struggled to find ways to help the Armenians understand the role of practical training in the preparation of students in applied professional education programs. The value of practice-based training in social work was aided tremendously by the hands on availability of the Armenian American social worker, the initiator of the original collaboration, who was in the country frequently for extended time. While in Armenia he identified and developed a number of U.S. type field work education sites for YSU social work students. In addition he worked with faculty to understand the importance of field work education and its role in making the program a success. To help everyone involved in the field education process understand their important roles he wrote and translated a field work manual for faculty, field work instructors and students. The manual explained and illustrated the field work education process. The availability of an on-site experienced social work practitioner knowledgeable in the language and culture was an essential component of the success of this project.

Initially the sociology faculty and others in the university were unconvinced of the value of practical training as an appropriate responsibility of a university and some wondered if such programs were more appropriate to a non-university setting. The UConn collaborators argued the value of university-based professional education and eventually were persuasive. More recently, YSU administrators told the authors that the model of practical training and international collaboration demonstrated by the Sociology and Social Work Department should be followed by other departments (Personal Communication, 2002). The Armenian University hopes that future collaboration with UConn will be broadened to other academic departments and disciplines.

While the social work education programs grew at the university, social service programs, both government programs and NGOs, flourished in the first decade of the new country's existence. Interestingly, social work in Armenia has developed along a similar path as happened in the United States one hundred years ago. For example, social workers have become part of many of the Armenian hospitals and schools just as happened in the U.S. In addition, a number of specialized community based social service NGOs have become a regular part of the landscape of resources in the new country. Several of the YSU faculty have founded and continue to provide leadership to a number of interesting and innovative social service NGOs. In this way the faculty are learning first hand about social work *practice*. Adding social service programs has been difficult since there is little money for new initiatives and still some misunderstanding among the general public about the value of professional helping services. Nonetheless, new programs are proliferating and the variety and quality of these programs are impressive. Many of these programs are supported by charitable donations from the diaspora and others interested in stabilizing the new republic through the introduction of an infrastructure of a civil society. Relatively small charitable contributions from the diaspora can support whole programs. While the cost of living has climbed significantly, salaries have not risen anywhere near as fast so a relatively small sum can support a number of staff. For example, a contribution of $250 can support a program for pregnant women that includes several staff for one month.

A variety of professional, self help and mutual aid activities emerged in the new Republic of Armenia. Many of these assisted refugees, earthquake survivors and others who had been displaced in the new economy. Often refugees, survivors and displaced persons banded together in formal and informal organizations to advocate for and protect their own interests. Currently, there are more than forty NGOs involved in refugee support and advocacy activities in Armenia (Alaverdyan, 2000). Some of the new NGOs were local branches of international organizations which were financially supported by outsiders. Much of this generosity came from the world wide diaspora. Some NGOs served all groups while others concentrated their resources on refugees, earthquake survivors or other displaced groups. In addition to direct services, NGOs also engaged in a variety of community development strategies to create services that would meet current and future needs. Still other NGOs concentrated on local and national educational services that informed the population, including government, of the needs and views of specific groups. Collectively the newly formed NGOs have played an important part in providing services, in promoting understanding and humane treatment of the population, and building the necessary infra-structure of a modern civil society. The NGOs have also had an important role in the development of social work in Armenia.

The development of government and NGO social service programs and the social work profession have grown together, and, in fact, are interdependent. More service programs created job opportunities for more social workers. Although not all of the new social workers were formally educated, some were trained in one or more short term training programs while others just began working with people. Currently Armenian social work is a mix of formally educated, trained and untrained practitioners. In an effort to increase the professionalism of social work the faculty initiated the first professional association. The Armenian Society of Social Scientists was founded by the sociology and social work faculties. The Armenian Association of Social Workers is a division within the larger Society. The professional association was created in order to advance the professionalism of social work. In addition to encouraging the formation of the social work association, the UConn has helped the larger association found a professional and scholarly journal *Social Transitions*. A UConn social work faculty member serves on the editorial review board. Several U.S. faculty have published in the new journal. Some financial support for the journal has been arranged through the collaboration. The UConn faculty hope that the social work association will soon turn its attention to the creation of the first code of ethics for social work in Armenia. An important aspect of the collaboration in the development of social work has been to insure that the profession develops in a way that is compatible with the Armenian culture. Cultural relevance is particularly important when thinking about values and ethics.

One of the most exciting elements of the collaboration has been funded travel opportunities for selected UConn MSW students who spend their spring break in Armenia working on projects in support of the development of social work. To date ten UConn students have traveled to Armenia. In 2000 two Armenian American students from UConn traveled to Armenia as a part of their field placement. Both were part of the diaspora. One of them had been raised in the Armenian culture. The other had an Armenian "ian" name but knew little else about her cultural heritage. Both returned from what they described as a life-altering experience. They worked on two projects. The first involved the development of a 50 minute video–*Beginning Where the Soviet Ends: The Story of the Development of Social Work in Armenia*. The video has had wide circulation in social work education and among the diaspora. The second project involved a series of eight focus groups with various subgroups of women in a Soviet-style planned community outside the capital city. The purpose of the focus groups was to understand the women's social service needs and to help women face the many problems associated with the dramatic transition in government and the economy which came as a result of the break up of the Soviet Union. The focus groups' data were analyzed and shared with local officials and published in *Social Transitions* (Humphreys and Simonian 2002).

The focus group method proved to be a particularly valid approach for capturing the experiences of women in Armenia, a group most affected by the dramatic transformations that occurred in the country. Women in Armenia have felt the brunt of the social, political and economic transformations that have taken place since Armenia became independent.

Like women everywhere, women in Armenia are the "rescuers of the family" since they are often the only adults in communities while men are away fighting wars or earning money (Van Wormer 1997).

Saulnier (1996) argues that "structural adjustment," the term she uses to refer to the movement from a planned central economy to one that is a free market system, affects women especially hard since they are the ones responsible for ensuring that families get along on whatever resources are available. The experiences of women are an important window into the well being of a society. The data from the focus groups tell an important story about the transitions in Armenia, particularly their effects on women and children as well as showing how women are coping and ultimately surviving in their new world.

The findings were many and important. None were more important than the finding that most of the participants were now living as single-parent mother-headed families because the husband/fathers were economic refugees, having left the community or country to find work in other areas. The most disturbing fact about this growing phenomenon is that some of the single parents had learned that their absent husbands were forming new families in their new place of residence. Thus, the loss of economic opportunity resulted in a dramatic growth in single-parent mother-headed families. The long term impact of these social changes are not yet well understood.

None of the other student travelers were of Armenian descent and yet they all experienced what they described as very significant experiences. Students have completed evaluations of several newly created social service programs, consulted with community leaders about new social service activities, visited and worked in refugee programs, met with students and faculty to exchange teaching and learning ideas and evaluated the technology capacity that could facilitate future collaborations. In many instances the U.S. students have maintained contact with those they met in Armenia. The collaboration between the two universities and social work faculties has been advanced and made richer by student experiences. A future hope of the collaboration is that sufficient funding can be found to support true international student exchanges with students from both programs regularly traveling to the other country.

In 2003, the authors initiated an innovative joint teaching assignment. Seven UConn and eleven YSU social work students completed a course titled "*Social Work and Social Welfare in the Second World.*" The course was taught using Web CT an electronic classroom that includes an e-mail and chat room features. The course was a comparative social welfare policy analysis with an emphasis on the context and substance of social welfare policy in Armenia and selected other newly independent republics formerly part of the Soviet Union. Working in cross national teams using Web CT students completed comparative policy analysis in three countries, Armenia, United States and one other country in the former Soviet Union. The course was carefully evaluated. Not surprising the major difficulties were unequal access to computers and the internet and language difficulties. Despite these difficulties the course will be taught again in the near future.

CONCLUSION

The development of social work and NGOs in Armenia have been influenced greatly by the needs of refugee populations and other persons who have been displaced by the new social and economic system. While the emerging patterns in Armenia are unique to its particular culture and time, it is interesting that the pattern in Armenia closely follows what happened in the United States more than one hundred years ago. In a similar way, the development of social work in Armenia replicated what happened in the United States, specifically the hiring of individual social workers to work in existing social institutions such as schools and hospitals and the evolution of the profession in these fields of practice. These developments occurred naturally and were not the result of any systematic plan or consultation with international collaborators.

While Armenian migration patterns have been similar to other countries in its link to social work and the creation of NGOs, they were unique because of the role that Armenians in the world wide diaspora have played in the affairs of the country both while it was a part of the Soviet Union and more recently after it became an independent country. The advent of social work as a profession and NGOs have occurred in many of the other newly independent countries of the former Soviet Union. However, the power and role of the Armenian diaspora has uniquely contributed to both the emergence of a free and independent Armenia and the development of social work as a new profession in the new republic.

Finally, the particular nature and forms of the collaboration with one school of social work in the United States and the newly created social work program in Armenia has many features which could serve as a model for others who wish to become involved in cross national collaboration.

REFERENCES

Ahearn, F.L. (1995). Displaced people. In Richard L. Edwards (Ed.) *Encyclopedia of Social Work*–19th edition. Washington, DC: NASW.

Alaverdyan, L. (2001). The problem of refugees and poverty reduction strategy in Armenia. www.worldbank.org/wbil/devdebates/ecal/alaveryan.pdf.

Balakian, P. (1997). *Black dog of fate: An American son uncovers his Armenian past.* New York: Broadway Books.

Davis, L. & Hagen, J. L. (1996). Stereotypes and stigma: What's changed for welfare mothers? *Affilia*, 11(3), 319-337.

Davis, L. & Srinivasan, M. (1995). Listening the to the voices of battered women: What helps them escape violence? *Affilia*, 10(1), 49-69.

Elektron.ettudeft.nl/~edo/armhist.html

Gareginian, A. (11/2001) AIM. (Armenian International Magazine), pp. 22-23.

Humanitarian Aid Corridor Act, HR1868, 104th Cong. (1995).

Humphreys, N.A. & Simonian, J. (2002) Women's voices from an artificial village. *Armenian Women*, 1(2).

Midgley, J. (1997). *Social welfare in global context.* Thousand Oaks, CA: Sage.

Roche, S. E. (1996). Messages from the NGO Forum on Women in Beijing 1995. *Affilia*, 11(4), 484-494.

Saulnier, C. F. (1996). *Feminist theories and social work: Approaches and applications.* New York: The Haworth Press.

Urwin, C. A. & Haynes, D. T. (1998). A reflexive model for collaboration: Empowering partnerships through focus groups. *Administration in Social Work*, 22(2), 23-39.

Van Wormer, K. (1997) *Social welfare: A world view.* Chicago: Nelson-Hall Publishers.

Strengthening the Link:
Social Work with Immigrants and Refugees and International Social Work

Lynne M. Healy

SUMMARY. Through exploration of definitional issues and current migration realities, this article discusses ways in which emphasis on the international dimensions of social work with immigrants and refugees offers opportunities to improve practice and to enhance the relevance of international social work to the profession. The international character of present day migration is illustrated through discussion of the transnational family and the economic and other relationships that tie immigrants to their countries of origin. The paper concludes with recommendations for increased cross-national professional collaboration. *[Article copies available for a fee from The Haworth Document Delivery Service: 1-800-HAWORTH. E-mail address: <docdelivery@haworthpress.com> Website: <http://www.HaworthPress.com> © 2004 by The Haworth Press, Inc. All rights reserved.]*

KEYWORDS. International social work, transnationals, immigrants, immigration, remittances

---

Lynne M. Healy, PhD, is Director, Center for International Social Work Studies, and Professor, School of Social Work, University of Connecticut.

[Haworth co-indexing entry note]: "Strengthening the Link: Social Work with Immigrants and Refugees and International Social Work." Healy, Lynne M. Co-published simultaneously in *Journal of Immigrant & Refugee Services* (The Haworth Social Work Practice Press, an imprint of The Haworth Press) Vol. 2, No. 1/2, 2004, pp. 49-67; and: *Immigrants and Social Work: Thinking Beyond the Borders of the United States* (ed: Diane Drachman, and Ana Paulino) The Haworth Social Work Practice Press, an imprint of The Haworth Press, Inc., 2001, pp. 49-67. Single or multiple copies of this article are available for a fee from The Haworth Document Delivery Service [1-800-HAWORTH, 9:00 a.m. - 5:00 p.m. (EST). E-mail address: docdelivery@haworthpress.com].

49

From its earliest conceptualizations, international social work has been intertwined with issues of migration and social work with immigrant and refugee populations. This paper will explore the commonalities, linkages and definitional tensions between the fields of social work with immigrants and refugees and international social work. Both historical and contemporary definitions and issues will be explored. I will argue that emphasis on the international dimensions of social work with immigrants and refugees offers opportunities to improve practice with these groups while enhancing the relevance of international social work to the social work profession.

Definitional issues will be addressed in detail, beginning with an examination of the history of the concept of international social work and its links to migration issues. To illustrate the international character of present day social work migration practice, the paper will discuss the growth in the phenomenon of the permanently transnational family; transnationalism will be further illustrated through a discussion of remittances–the economic transfers made to family members abroad–and a brief consideration of the global context of immigration policy. The paper will close with a recommendation for increased cross-national professional collaboration between sending and receiving countries to improve migration practice in the context of an uncertain future.

DEFINITIONS OF INTERNATIONAL SOCIAL WORK

Definitions in Historical Perspective

The international character of practice with immigrants was recognized early in the history of social work. In a call for more social service involvement in migration research, a committee chaired by Edith Abbott reported: "It (the field of human migration) includes large questions of public policy, involving issues of national prosperity and human rights . . . It presents problems that reach beyond the frontiers of any one nation, and many of its research problems are of international importance and demand international co-operation for their solution" (Human Migration as a Field of Research, 1927, p. 258). The need for knowledge and skill in international casework to serve migrants was discussed at the First International Conference of Social Work, held in Paris in 1928. The presenter drew attention to the "lack of understanding of the international aspects of these problems" (deBacourt, 1929, p. 426). A few years later, it was described in an article in the 3rd edition of the

U.S. *Social Work Yearbook*: "international social casework problems arise in public and private welfare agencies because of the migration of individuals and families to and from the United States" (Warren, 1935, p. 214). Beginning in the next volume of the *Yearbook* in 1937, international casework was subsumed under the definition of international social work as one of three types of activity making up this field of practice: international social casework, international conferences on social work, and international efforts to address problems in the fields of health, labor and protection of women and children (Warren, 1937), a definition later expanded to include other types of international assistance (Warren, 1939).

Recognition of the complexities of problems faced by immigrant families and the concomitant need for broad international knowledge on the part of practitioners were evident in these early articles, as the following example illustrates: The family problems presented are associated with or grow out of the experience of migration, often many years later. All members of a family rarely migrate together. The father or husband generally precedes the other members of the family. Families are thus separated for temporary or longer periods of time. Restrictive immigration and naturalization laws and the act of migration itself interrupt the natural rhythm of family life. Civil and social rights and the benefits of social institutions are unavailable for migrant families during the period of alienage until citizenship in the country of immigration is secured by all members of the family. Deficiencies in civil status thus combine with the handicaps of foreignness and the environmental and personal hazards of family life to present problems for international social case work service (Warren, 1941, p. 271).Warren continues on to discuss the need for information about the cultural backgrounds of the countries from which migrants originate in order to provide adequate services in child welfare, hospitals, the criminal justice system, and other institutions. Thus, in the early part of the 20th century, social work experts recognized the important international dimensions of practice with immigrants and refugees including differences in national cultures, human rights, family separation across borders, immigration laws and foreign policies. Furthermore, knowledge in these areas was recognized as important for social workers in mainstream practice in child welfare, health care, and criminal justice, not just for immigration specialists.

The need for international knowledge in service to refugee and migrant families became even more evident during World War II as large numbers of persons were displaced. In her article on international social work, Larned explained: "Local case workers were baffled because

these situations had roots in two or more countries and were complicated not only by distance and separation of families, but also by differences in cultural backgrounds and attitudes of the individuals concerned,
differences in national laws affecting family relationships and citizenship, and differences in the concepts of social care" (1945, p. 191).

Throughout the 1920s, 1930s and 1940s, then, social work recognized the special knowledge and practice demands of work with international migrants and often conceptualized this practice as a component
of international social work. While a detailed account of shifts in conceptualization of international social work is not warranted here, in brief,
changes were evident beginning in the 1950s. A study undertaken in the
mid-1950s by a working committee of the Council on Social Work Education stands out. After reviewing multiple definitions of the term international social work including those that addressed work with refugees
and immigrants, the Committee broke away from the Warren and
Larned definitions and opted for a very narrow definition of international
social work focusing on work for intergovernmental or international
agencies (Stein, 1957). In the words of the Committee report: "It was
the consensus of our sub-committee that the term 'international social
work' should properly be confined to programs of social work of international scope, such as those carried on by intergovernmental agencies,
chiefly those of the U.N.; governmental; or nongovernmental agencies
with international programs" (Stein, 1957, p. 3). This was followed in
the 1970s and 1980s by relative isolationism within the profession in
North America before a resurgence of interest in internationalism in the
1990s (Healy, 1995; Healy, 1999).

While many factors have contributed to the resurgence of interest in
international social work, it is likely that the expansion of international
migration and the growth of the foreign born population in the U.S. and
many other countries are particularly significant. In the United States,
for example, the 1930 census revealed that 11.3% of the population was
foreign born and that the foreign born together with their children comprised almost one-third of the total population (Warren, 1935). After
several decades of steep decline, the foreign born proportion of the population has again grown to 10.4% as of 2000, close to the 11.3% level of
1930. The growth of immigrant and refugee populations has had a world-
wide impact. Guest workers from Southern Europe and North Africa
have become long term residents in Northern Europe at the same time
that refugee populations have increased, turning previously homogenous countries such as Denmark and Sweden into multicultural ones.

Imported laborers work in many of the Gulf States and in countries such as Cote d'Ivoire that hosts as many as 2 million workers from neighboring Burkina Faso (U.S. Department of State, 2001). Developing countries, too, experience the impact of refugee flows; while refugee resettlement programs in Europe and North America draw considerable attention, most of the world's refugees flee to neighboring countries. In 1996, for example, there were almost 2 million refugees from tiny Rwanda in the neighboring countries of Zaire (now Congo), Burundi, Tanzania and Uganda (UNDP, 1996); the recent flow of Afghan refugees to Pakistan is actually a continuation of a long-term refugee problem in the area. Thus, at the beginning of the 21st century, many if not most countries of the world are faced with significant international populations within their borders. Shifts in the size and diversity of foreign born populations may well shape the conceptualization of both international social work and social work with immigrants and refugees.

Contemporary Definitional Issues

Contemporary dictionary definition of the term "international" supports a link to service to refugees and immigrants. According to the *Random House Webster's College Dictionary* (1995), international can refer to any of the following: "between or among two or more nations, . . . of or pertaining to two or more nations or their citizens, . . . pertaining to the relations between nations, . . . having members or activities in several nations, . . . transcending national boundaries or viewpoints" (p. 704). Work with immigrants clearly pertains to the citizens of two or more nations, and the field of immigration practice and policy indeed transcends national boundaries.

Building on this, a recent action-focused definition of international social work, identified the first of four components of the field as "social work competence in internationally related aspects of domestic social work practice and professional advocacy" (Healy, 2001, p. 7). While there are other aspects of internationally related domestic practice, it is the international movement of people that has changed social agency caseloads and affected social work practice in many countries, especially the United States. Therefore work with international migrant populations is the most important component of internationally related domestic practice.

Some contemporary writers disagree with the inclusion of work with international populations under the international social work umbrella.

Nagy and Falk (2000) suggest that although "some definitions of international social work appear to include social work practice with immigrants, refugees or ethnic minorities, in the social worker's own country" (p. 53) this type of practice should "be distinguished from social work across national borders" (p. 53). They argue that the emphasis in practice with refugees and immigrants should be on inter-cultural or multi-cultural practice, rather than on international social work. This author agrees that the multicultural perspective has dominated recent social work practice with immigrants and refugees in the U.S., but to its detriment. The result has been diminished application of relevant international knowledge and understanding to provision of services to immigrants and refugees and severely limited capacity to engage in successful policy advocacy on migration issues.

Two important elements differentiate social work with immigrants and refugees from multicultural work with domestic minority groups. The first and most critical is the migration experience. As clearly described by Drachman (1992), effective social work with immigrants and refugees requires knowledge of their country of origin experiences, the factors that led to the decision to migrate, their transit experiences, and resettlement. These fall primarily in the arena of international knowledge. Phases of the process are governed by a complex set of national and international laws on refugee movements, resettlement, entitlements and immigration, by the foreign policies of the nations involved, and by international policy on human rights.

The second element is the ongoing transnational nature of the migration phenomenon. At the micro level, this is reflected in the transnational family; families of many if not most immigrants are now transnational families in that members and relationships span borders throughout the family life cycle. A recent obituary in the Hartford *Courant* illustrates a not unusual case: the deceased was born in rural Jamaica and had lived in the U.S. in both Connecticut and Florida. He left 5 siblings, two in England, one in the U.S., and two in Jamaica. His seven children reside in Canada, the U.S. and Jamaica (April 26, 2001). One can imagine the life of this family and the frequent exchange of communications, money and people across the borders of four countries. In these exchanges, the family would have been touched by laws and economic policies of multiple countries and perhaps, of international organizations. Social workers involved with transnational families face many knowledge demands beyond those of cross-cultural or multicultural social work. Transnationalism also has significant effects at the macro level of national economic development policy and foreign affairs. Understanding the transnational relationships that affect and are affected by migration equips social work to improve practice and to engage in appropriate policy advocacy. These points will be elaborated below.

THE TRANSNATIONAL FAMILY: THE NEW FACE OF INTERNATIONAL MIGRATION

Family Relationships

Increasingly, immigrants are part of families that remain transnational. In some, family members are separated for long periods of time or even permanently by international migration. Others may live simultaneously in two countries, traveling back and forth between employment and family, without or without legal sanction. Still others, long resettled, plan to return some day to their country of origin, and prepare for another round of leaving, transit and resettlement–perhaps creating new family separations in the process.

In each of these situations, family members maintain relationships through communications, exchange of money and goods across borders, and sometimes, visitation and plans for additional family members to immigrate or emigrate. Issues of custody, divorce, support and child visitation are more complicated when parties live in different countries, creating special challenges for social workers. There is a specialized agency, International Social Service, that provides intercountry casework services for cross-national permanency planning, custody evaluations, counseling on inter-country marriages and divorces, tracing of separated family members, child support, and inter-country adoption in 75 countries (see www.iss-ssi.org for more information). However, it serves a relatively small percent of intercountry cases. Most are left to social workers in local immigrant and refugee service agencies and to mainstream social workers in child welfare services, schools, hospitals, and mental health agencies; these workers usually lack specialized training in intercountry work and may fail to recognize the international dimensions of their clients' problems.

More common than intercountry custody, divorce and visitation are the issues raised by family reunification following long periods of separation for social workers in receiving countries while social workers in sending countries deal with the impact of long separations on children. A common pattern of immigration is for a parent to immigrate first, leaving minor children in the care of spouse, grandparents, or others in the home country. Those left behind are sent for once the parent is financially secure and immigration regulations have been satisfied. By then, the period of separation may have stretched to three to five years or even more. Meanwhile, social workers in the sending countries must deal with children who feel abandoned, who are sometimes left in unsatisfactory care situations, and who may lose their motivation for school and other activities as they wait for what they believe will be imminent emigration. In the receiving countries, social workers encounter children and parents who struggle to build relationships after years of separation and often, very little personal communication, while the newly arrived cope with their new environment. That reunification often happens in the early teen years further complicates family adjustment.

Crawford-Brown and Rattray (2001) described a difficult set of cases which they labeled "barrel children." It is common for immigrants from the Caribbean to send home goods to family members, commonly shipping them in barrels. Some of these goods go to the children left behind, usually with relatives. Crawford-Brown, however, documented that some teenage children are left on their own by emigrating parents; the parents send barrels of goods for the children to sell to support themselves. The negative side of the story is of course that children are sometimes physically and emotionally abandoned through immigration, with parents retaining only the role of financial support. Financial support of children and other relatives is, on the other hand, a dominant factor in the transnational phenomenon of migration, as will be addressed in detail below. The issue of remittances has been selected as an example to demonstrate the international dimension of migration at the micro and macro levels, and its impact on social work.

Remittances: Transnational Family Economics

The transnational character of immigration and its impact at family and national levels is clearly demonstrated by remittances–money sent back to family members in the home country by migrants abroad. As described in a recent report by the Inter-American Development Bank, "as the scale of migration has increased in recent years and the growth of remittances has accelerated dramatically, the social and economic impact of this phenomenon now transcends family relationships and is drawing national and international attention" (2001, p. 4). The report estimates that immigrants in North America sent $20 billion dollars to their home countries in Latin America and the Caribbean alone in 2000 (IADB, 2001, p. 6). This represents the accumulation of millions of individual transactions, with the typical migrant sending home about $250 at a time, eight to ten times a year (IADB, p. 6). The reader is reminded that these figures only address the Western hemisphere; globally, the total flow of remittances was estimated at over $71 billion in 1990, a figure that has undoubtedly grown since then (Meyers, 1998).

At the macro level, it is now recognized that remittances are essential to the receiving economies. In Jamaica, the value of remittances is second only to tourism as a source of foreign exchange (PIOJ,1999) and is 35 times more than the amount of foreign aid received (IADB, 2001). Thus, many Jamaicans look to their relatives abroad to help make ends meet; the money received and spent undoubtedly does more to aid the local economy than foreign aid. The significant economic impact is not limited to Jamaica. In five other countries in the region, remittances account for 10% or more of the Gross Domestic Product (GDP): Haiti, Nicaragua, El Salvador, the Dominican Republic and Ecuador (IADB, p. 6). So important are the impacts of these individual efforts combined that they are recognized parts of some countries' foreign policy efforts. One scholar notes that in a recent visit to the U.S. by the President of El Salvador, he requested an increased number of work permits for Salvadoran immigrants to enter or remain in the U.S. in order to help rebuild El Salvador after several natural disasters as "the increased earnings that legally authorized workers could remit would far outweigh the likely foreign aid that would be forthcoming" (Martin, 2001, p. 4). As a final example, Mexico, with an estimated eight million native born Mexicans now residing in the U.S., is the single largest recipient of remittances in Latin America, receiving almost $7 billion in 1999, almost equaling the amount earned from tourism (IADB, 2001).

Emigration clearly has some negative effects on developing countries as it is often the skilled workers who are most likely to leave ("Emigration: Outward Bound," 2002). Understanding the role of remittances clarifies why sending countries may have an interest in maintaining high levels of emigration nonetheless. Emigration is an outlet for areas with high unemployment and limited income-generating possibilities; the remittances received from those who leave represent a significant force in their home country economies, aiding family survival at the micro level, providing at least consumer-level economic stimulus, and assisting with balance of payments at the macro level. A recent study of coping strategies of minimum wage workers in Jamaica showed that "the main support for all groups came from relatives and friends living overseas" (Henry-Lee, Chevannes, Clarke and Ricketts, 2000, p. 26);

47% of domestic helpers, 78% of free zone workers, and 64% of security guards received money from relatives or friends who live abroad.

While remittances tend to subside after one or two generations of immigrants, the new realities of global interdependence and increased transnationalism strengthen the ties of immigrants to their home communities and may lengthen the period of remittances. Martin notes that the increase in transnationalism is due in part to "the transportation and communications revolution that makes it easier to move and keep contact with one's home community"; "migrants can now live at one and the same time in two different countries" by maintaining constant contact, visits, and sending resources home (2001, p. 2).

The practice of remittances obviously has a significant impact on immigrant families in their new country of residence. Social workers need to be aware of this often hidden financial obligation assumed by immigrant families. Both the policy and personal impacts remain under-studied. Martin points out that while remittances obviously benefit poor families in developing countries, "it means that the poorest residents of the U.S. and other wealthy countries are bearing the brunt of assisting people in developing countries. Latin American migrants tend to have low incomes, often living in poverty, yet they remit billions of dollars to their home countries" (2001, p. 5). Client immigrant families may make decisions that puzzle their social worker–for example, not pursuing advanced training or working multiple jobs, seemingly failing to fulfill some family responsibilities such as spending time with their children. During the resettlement phase of work with refugees, their sense of obligation to send remittances to their home country conflicts with the priority on rapid self-sufficiency in resettlement policy, posing a dilemma for social work. A resettlement worker recounted a case in which a man from the Northern Sudan, being resettled in South Dakota, was sending money home to his wife in Sudan, although he did not have enough to pay his bills or even buy adequate food for himself. In keeping with agency and indeed national policy, the social worker repeatedly told him not to send money home until he was fully self-sufficient. Unless the social worker has knowledge of the international picture of immigration, he or she is likely to have an incomplete understanding of family responsibilities as viewed by the immigrant–and indeed, by his or her country of origin. Thus, the international perspective that transcends national boundaries and points of view is important.

IMMIGRATION POLICY:
TRANSCENDING NATIONAL BOUNDARIES

Immigration policy is inherently international policy, emanating from broad agreements of international law and refined by each nation's foreign policy imperatives. Social workers' ability to help immigrants and refugees is aided or, more often, constrained by these official global and foreign policies. Understanding of immigration and refugee policy is necessary to properly advise clients on procedures and entitlements and to allow social workers to advocate for more humane and family-oriented immigration policies in their own country and globally.

At the global level, the right to emigrate–to leave one's country–is viewed as an important human right. Article 13 of the Universal Declaration of Human Rights states: "Everyone has the right to leave any country, including his own, and to return to his country" (1948). However, no corresponding right to enter or immigrate is recognized in international law. Other than the protections for officially recognized refugees, this policy mismatch leaves those who wish to emigrate in an insecure position. Refugee policy, too, begins with the internationally recognized definition of a refugee and official recognition of status by the United Nations High Commission on Refugees. Individual country decisions to grant refugee status are governed at least as much by foreign policy as by humanitarian concerns.

The inherent unfairness of immigration policies is troubling to many social workers and others. Indeed, Isbister wrote that in various ways, immigration policy is "inherently immoral" (1996, p. 229). The recent deportation provisions in U.S. Immigration law provide an example of policy of questionable morality and significant international impact. The 1996 Illegal Immigration Reform and Immigrant Responsibility Act and the Anti-Terrorism and Effective Death Penalty Act contained draconian deportation provisions that have had significant national and international impact at both family and societal levels. These acts: increased the number of deportable offenses to include family violence offenses and some fairly minor crimes by reclassifying them retroactively as felonies; called for deportation for offenses committed 20 or more years ago, even if when committed the offense would not have qualified as a felony; and completely eliminated the appeals process (Ward, 1999). Furthermore, those deported are permanently barred from the United States. Deportations have soared since the laws went into effect (Rich, 2000).

In countries of origin that have received increased numbers of deportees since 1996, these have been of two types. Migrants convicted of serious drug and violent offenses were deported home often without warning to officials, unleashing a wave of crime in their home countries (Maxwell, 1990; Guyana Online, 2001). When governments protested, their protests were largely ignored. The U.S. government recently halted issuing visas for citizens of Guyana to retaliate against the Guyana government for refusing to accept criminal deportees, demonstrating again that immigration policy is critical bi-national foreign policy (Guyana Online, 2001). The other type of deportees are those who have committed minor offenses, perhaps years ago when they were young; these deportees may have emigrated at an early age and have few current ties in their home country and therefore no means of support. "Because most of them have lived almost all their adult lives in North America and are more the products of those societies than they are of Guyana, they are in a very real sense strangers in the land of their birth" (Guyana Online, 2001). Obviously, remittances from those deported cease, affecting their families as well. Thus, countries with very limited resources for law enforcement and high rates of unemployment and poverty are forced or pressured to accept back criminal emigres and others with no prospects for jobs or income.

The domestic impact in the U.S. has also been severe. Marital partners have been separated by sudden deportation, and parents have been separated from their U.S. citizen children, sometimes leaving families with no means of support and children without parental supervision (Hedges, 2001). As the law calls for no appeal and permanent ban from reentering the U.S., the separation is permanent unless the children move to their parent's country of origin. Both the personal and fiscal impact of these policies has been locally and internationally harmful.

Social work responsibilities in this arena begin with adequate knowledge of immigration policy in order to avoid doing harm. In some cases, well-meaning social workers advised clients to seek citizenship to remain eligible for the entitlements that were cut off for legal immigrants in another of the 1996 policies. Unfortunately, it was during citizenship application processes that many of the deportees were "uncovered" as prior offenders. Secondly, the professional needs knowledge of the global interactions of immigration policy in order to formulate sound campaigns for reform, both nationally and cross-nationally. These obligations are recognized in the NASW policy statement on Immigrants and Refugees that reads, in part: "Social workers must continue to advocate for family reunification and sanctuary from persecution and insist that due process and fundamental human rights be upheld for immigrants and refugees. The profession must promote greater education and awareness at all levels of the dynamics of U.S. and other countries' foreign policies on immigration and refugee resettlement" (NASW, 2000, p. 176).

PROSPECTS FOR THE FUTURE

International Collaboration in Immigrant Work

Conceptualizing work with immigrants and refugees as international social work and accepting the need for international knowledge can lead to more than an understanding of the transnational family and the global policy context. It may also open up new avenues for intervention. There is considerable untapped potential for international collaboration in social work. Cross-national social work collaboration to smooth the immigration and resettlement processes would be an excellent place to begin such efforts. This is especially true in those areas which receive steady influx of immigrants from particular countries. Working together, social workers in the sending and receiving countries could develop interventions to assist in the leaving and resettlement processes. The process could begin with information sharing about the needs and problems experienced on both sides of the immigration journey. Information about schools, expectations, and other living conditions in the destination areas could be sent to social workers in the countries where children wait to join their parents. One social worker proposed making a video-tape showing school and typical home life, with brief interviews of immigrant children. Social workers in source countries would use such a tape in groups for "children in waiting." Social workers in immigrant-receiving areas might use their knowledge of immigration patterns and children's needs coupled with insights gained through communication with colleagues in the sending country to reach out to immigrants and offer pre-reunification counseling or information sessions to advise parents on the need to stay in personal and emotional contact with their children and to prepare them to cope with the usually unanticipated stresses of reunification (Crawford-Brown and Rattrey, 2001).

Cross-national communication between social workers on a continuing basis could provide cross-cultural consultation to assist social workers in serving immigrant families and meeting the special needs of the transnational family. Finally, such collaborations can be of particular benefit in resolving those cases requiring inter-country casework, such as custody issues, child placement in cases of parental death, deportation, or other causes; preparation for return migration of elders, and other cases involving bi-national legal/social service matters.

The ease of email communications and the possibilities offered by video and web-based technologies for information exchange, outreach and education should not be underestimated.

Post-September 11 Trends in International Aspects of Migration

The aftermath of the terrorist attacks on the U.S. mainland in September, 2001 make long term projections about immigration and about professional and societal openness to emphasis on its international dimensions difficult, not only in the U.S. but in many other countries. Some of the changes anticipated will affect social work practice with immigrants and refugees; most will certainly increase the need for international understanding. Early indications are that many countries are slowing the issuing of visas and exploring ways to protect their borders from terrorists, actions that may impede normal immigration and complicate the lives of members of transnational families (Keep America's Gates Open, 2001; Government of Canada, 2001). These changes are likely to mean slower reunifications and restrictions on visitation of family members who remain separated. Deportations may also increase, with Middle Eastern immigrants a special target. In the U.S., several areas of immigration policy relief have been shelved, most notably the proposal to regularize some undocumented immigrants from Mexico and others to provide relief from deportation provisions of the 1996 laws (Brownstein, 2001; Pena, 2001).

A retreat to isolationism, however, does not look likely. Instead, the events heightened awareness of the need for international knowledge and understanding. Most writers also believe that any downturn in immigration rates will be temporary. The pressures creating high emigration from source countries continue to be strong. In fact, the economic fallout from the September 11 events have increased the push factors for immigration through their negative impact on the economies of developing countries. According to the World Bank, "ripples from the September 11 attacks will be felt across all the world's regions, particularly in countries dependent on tourism, remittances from populations living overseas, and foreign investment" ("Poverty to Rise . . ." 2001, p. 2). The travel and tourism industry has been particularly hit hard; thus in Jamaica, for example, where pre-September 11th unemployment rate was

16% (Thomas, 2001) unemployment in the tourist sector and businesses that supply the tourist sector is soaring as reservations are cancelled. In St. Lucia, the drop in tourist reservations for winter 2002 was so severe that the Club Med resort decided not to open for the season (Ballve, 2002). Overall, the World Bank reported that 65% of vacations booked for the Caribbean had been cancelled as of October 1, 2001. The impact on these economies that rely on tourism as their chief source of revenue has been devastating. The World Bank further estimated that as a result of the terrorist attacks, 10 million more people in developing countries could be pushed below the poverty line of $1 per day ("Poverty to Rise" 2001). Coupled with possible reductions in remittances that have cushioned the effects of poor local economic opportunities, pressures for emigration are high ("Latin American migrants in the United States sending less money home," 2001). Thus, understood in its global context, the aftermath of September 11 terrorist attacks has created both increased pressures for high immigration as economic opportunities diminish in countries of origin and increased resistance to the admittance of immigrants in many countries of destination. The long term impact may well be increases in immigration by those economically dislocated by these events–possibly through extra-legal channels. In an earlier document, the government of Jamaica explained: "Given that the pressures for emigration are high in Jamaica, especially since our labour force continues to increase, undocumented or irregular migration is expected to continue" (Planning Institute of Jamaica, 1995, p. 44).

CONCLUSION:
IS SOCIAL WORK WITH IMMIGRANTS
AND REFUGEES INTERNATIONAL SOCIAL WORK?

In conclusion, a return to the original question of the paper is in order. First, it may be useful to remember the insights of our professional "ancestors" who recognized the links between local and global events and the human rights and civil liberties elements of migration that are so relevant today. But, regardless of the historical links between migration practice and international social work, contemporary social work should renew the emphasis only if there is clear benefit to one or both knowledge areas. For international social work, work with immigrants and refugee populations provides the clearest and most concrete example of the necessity and applicability of international knowledge to social work. It makes the importance of international knowledge understandable in any society affected by international migration–a near universal phenomenon at the beginning of the 21st century. In countries with high levels of immigration or emigration, this inclusion also extends to all social workers the imperative for international knowledge. Rather than an esoteric specialty of a few, international knowledge is essential for competent social work in a country where one in ten inhabitants is an immigrant. The transnational family makes this as essential in countries with high rates of emigration. Furthermore, inclusion of practice with immigrants within international social work demonstrates the links between domestic and global issues, lending support to the argument that there is no such thing as purely domestic/local social work in the 21st century. Thus, development of the field of international social work is strengthened through linking it to practice with immigrants and refugees.

The benefits to the field of social work with immigrants and refugees may be more compelling and hopefully have been addressed in the preceding pages. Inclusion of international knowledge in practice with immigrants and refugees should improve practice by equipping social workers to understand the pre-migration, migration and resettlement phases of their clients' journeys (Drachman,1992) and preparing them to work with the ongoing transnational family issues faced by their clients. Only through knowledge of the international dimensions of immigration can social workers address the policy issues of work with migrants, including the impacts on sending countries. Finally, recognition of the international nature of immigration work may unleash the largely unexplored potential of cross-national collegial work to improve service to migrant populations.

Therefore, as stated by NASW, "social workers must give consideration to the global dynamic of immigration" (2000, p. 175). In recognizing the important linkages between international social work and social work with immigrants and refugees, both areas of social work will be strengthened.

REFERENCES

Ballve, M. (2002). Hotels Empty, Workers Idle. *Hartford Courant.* January 5, pp. E1, E8.
Brownstein, R. (2001). Green light, red light: Is the push to liberalize immigration policy a casualty of the surprise terrorist attacks on September 11? *The American Prospect.* 12:20, pp. 28- (obtained full text through InfoTrac).

Crawford-Brown, C.P.J. and Rattray, J.M. (2001). "Parent Child Relationships in Caribbean Families" in N. Boyd Webb (ed.) *Culturally Diverse Parent-Child and Family Relationships*. New York: Columbia University Press, pp. 107-32.

Debacourt, F. (1929). The need for international case work for migrants. in *Proceedings of the First International Conference of Social Work 1928*. Volume 2, Paris, International Conference of Social Work, pp. 416-432.

Drachman, D. (1992). A stage-of-migration framework for service to immigrant populations. *Social Work*. 37:1, 68-72.

"Emigration: Outward Bound" (2002). *The Economist*, Vol. 364, Number 8292 (September 26-October 4, 2002), pp. 24-26.

Government of Canada. (2001). Strengthened immigration measures to counter terrorism. News release, October 12, 2001. www.cic.gc.ca/english/press/01/0119-pre.html Accessed Jan. 4, 2002.

Guyana Online. (2001), Meeting public concerns over the deportee influx. 11/21/01. <www.guyanaonline.net/c-news/index> Accessed January 16, 2002.

Healy, L. (2001). *International Social Work: Professional Action in an Interdependent World*. New York: Oxford University Press.

Healy, L. (1999). International social work curriculum in historical perspective. in C.S. Ramanathan and R.J. Link, *All Our Futures: Principles and Resources for Social Work Practice in a Global Era*. Belmont, CA: Brooks/Cole, pp. 14-29.

Healy, L. (1995). Comparative and international overview. in T.D. Watts, D. Elliott, and N.S. Mayadas (Eds). *International handbook on social work education*. Westport, CT: Greenwood Press, pp. 421-439.

Hedges, C. (2001). Spousal deportation, Family ruin as breadwinners are exiled. *The New York Times*. January 10.

Henry-Lee, A., Chevannes, B., Clarke, M., and Ricketts, S. (2000). An assessment of the standard of living and coping strategies of workers in selected occupations who earn a minimum wage. Kingston, Jamaica: Policy Development Unit, Planning Institute of Jamaica.

Human migration as a field of research. (1927). *Social Service Review*. 1:2, 258-269.

Inter-American Development Bank (2001), Remittances to Latin America and the Caribbean: Comparative Statistics. Multilateral Investment Fund (May). accessed from www.iadb.org Accessed January 3, 2002.

International Social Service, (2002). Intercountry casework. <www.iss-ssi.org>. Accessed January 14, 2002.

Isbister, J. (1996). *The Immigration Debate: Remaking America*. West Hartford, CT: Kumarian Press.

Keep America's gates open, just watch them better. (2001). *Business Week*. Nov. 19, 13758. p. 72EU8. Obtained full text through InfoTrac OneFile.

Larned, R. (1945). International social work. in R.H. Kurz, ed., *Social Work Yearbook 1945*. New York: Russell Sage Foundation, 188-194.

Latin American migrants in the United States sending less money home in wake of September 11 attacks (2001). Press Release, December 17, 2001, Inter-American Development Bank. <www.iadb.org/exr/PRENSA/2001/cp23601E.htm>. Accessed January 8, 2002.

Martin, S.F. (2001). Remittance Flows and Impact. Paper prepared for the Remittances as a Development Tool Regional Conference, Inter-American Development Bank. Institute for the Study of International Migration, Georgetown University. www. iadb.org Accessed January 3, 2002.

Maxwell, J.A. (1990). Development of social welfare services and the field of social work in Jamaica. Paper presented at the Caribbean Conference for Social Workers, Paramaribo, Surinam.

Meyers, D.W. (1998). Migrant remittances to Latin America: Reviewing the literature. Working Paper: Inter-American Dialogue and the Tomas Rivera Policy Institute. May, 1998. Available at: www.iadialog.org/meyers.html Accessed January 7, 2002.

Nagy, G. and Falk, D. (2000). Dilemmas in international and cross-cultural social work education. *International Social Work*. 43:1, 49-60.

National Association of Social Workers (2000). Immigrants and refugees. in *Social Work Speaks*. Washington, D.C.: NASW Press, pp. 170-177.

Obituary. (2001) *The Hartford Courant*. Thursday, April 26, p. B6.

Pena, M. (2001). Immigration policy another victim of terrorist attacks. Agencia Efe S.A., Spain, September 17. Accessed through Comtext news (www.comtexnews. com) via InfoTrac.

Planning Institute of Jamaica (PIOJ). (1999). *Economic and Social Survey Jamaica 1998*. Kingston, Jamaica: author.

Planning Institute of Jamaica (PIOJ). (1995). *National Plan of Action on Population and Development Jamaica 1995-2015*. Kingston, Jamaica: Population Unit, PIOJ.

"Poverty to rise in wake of terrorist attacks in US." (2001, Oct. 1). *DevNews: The World Bank's Daily Webzine*. Washington, D.C.: World Bank. www.worldbank. org/developmentnew/stories/html/100101a.htm Accessed January 14, 2002.

Random House Webster's College Dictionary. (1995). New York: Random House.

Rich, E. (2000). Deportations soar under rigid law. *The Hartford Courant*. Vol. CLXII, No. 282. Sunday, October 8, pp. A1, A8, A9.

Stein, H. (1957). An international perspective in the social work curriculum. Paper presented at the Annual Meeting of the Council on Social Work Education, Los Angeles, CA, January, 1957.

Thomas, D. (2001). Jamaica: Economic Situation and Prospects. www.iadb.org/regions/ re3/sep/ja-sep Accessed January 15, 2002.

United Nations (1948). Universal declaration of human rights. New York: U.N. Department of Public Information or www.unhchr.org.ch/

United Nations Development Program (1996). *Human Development Report 1996*. New York: Oxford University Press.

United States Department of State. (2001). Background Note: Cote d'Ivoire. Bureau of African Affairs, November, 2001. *www.state.gov/p/af/ci/iv/* Accessed October 16, 2002.

Ward, C.A. (1999). Consequences of United State Immigration Policy: A Caribbean Perspective. Washington, D.C.: National Coalition on Caribbean Affairs.

Warren, G.L. (1935). International social casework. in F.S. Hall, ed. *Social Work Yearbook 1935*. New York: Russell Sage Foundation, 214-216.

Warren, G.L. (1937) International social work. in R.H. Kurz, ed. *Social Work Yearbook 1937*. New York: Russell Sage Foundation, 224-227.

Warren, G.L. (1939). International social work. in R.H. Kurz, ed. *Social Work Yearbook 1939*. New York: Russell Sage Foundation, 192-196.
Warren, G.L. (1941). International social work. in R.H. Kurz, ed. *Social Work Yearbook 1941*. New York: Russell Sage Foundation, 270-276.

FOR FURTHER READING AND RESEARCH

Drachman, D. (1992), A stage of migration framework for service to immigrant populations. *Social Work* 37:1, 68-72.
Healy, L. (2001). *International Social Work: Professional Action in an Interdependent World*. New York: Oxford University Press. Chapter 1: International Social Work: Why Is It Important and What Is It? and Chapter 9: International/Domestic Practice Interface.
Human migration as a field of research. (1927). *Social Service Review* 1:2, 258-269.
Immigrants and Refugees. (2000). *Social Work Speaks*. Compilation of NASW Policy Statements, Washington, DC: NASW Press.
International Policy on Migration; International Policy on Refugees; International Policy on Displaced Persons. *Policy Papers*. Berne, Switzerland: International Federation of Social Workers. (available at www.ifsw.org).

Resources on Social/Economic Conditions in Other Countries

Human Development Report. Annual. New York: United Nations Development Program (www.undp.org). Paper copy published by Oxford University Press, New York.
State of the World's Refugees. Annual. Geneva: United Nations High Commission on Refugees. (www.unhcr.ch) Paper copy published by Oxford University Press, New York.
World Development Report Annual. Washington, DC: The World Bank. (www.world bank.org).

Useful Websites on International Populations and on Remittances

Institute for the Study of International Migration, Georgetown University:
Inter-American Development Bank: <www.iadb.org>
Inter-American Dialogue: <www.iadialog.org>
International Social Service: <www.iss-ssi.org>
United Nations High Commission on Refugees: <www.unhcr.ch>

Neither Here Nor There:
Puerto Rican Circular Migration

Gregory Acevedo

SUMMARY. Since 1917 all Puerto Ricans, whether island- or mainland-born, are United States citizens. Physical proximity and relatively affordable transportation encourages Puerto Rican migration to the mainland United States. Puerto Rican migration takes three forms: the "one- way migrants," who move permanently to the mainland; the "return migrants" who migrate to the mainland but after many years return to the island and reestablish residence; and the "circular migrants" who migrate back and forth between the island and the mainland spending substantial periods of residence in both places. The following analysis emphasizes the conditions that instigate the departure of Puerto Rican migrants from both the island and the mainland, and discusses the implications of Puerto Rican circular migration for social work and the provision of social welfare programs and services. *[Article copies available for a fee from The Haworth Document Delivery Service: 1-800-HAWORTH. E-mail address: <docdelivery@haworthpress.com> Website: <http://www.HaworthPress.com> © 2004 by The Haworth Press, Inc. All rights reserved.]*

KEYWORDS. Puerto Rico, Puerto Rican migration, migration, immigration, circular migration

Gregory Acevedo, PhD, is Assistant Professor of Social Work, School of Social Administration, Temple University.

[Haworth co-indexing entry note]: "Neither Here Nor There: Puerto Rican Circular Migration." Acevedo, Gregory. Co-published simultaneously in *Journal of Immigrant & Refugee Services* (The Haworth Social Work Practice Press, an imprint of The Haworth Press) Vol. 2, No. 1/2, 2004, pp. 69-85; and: *Immigrants and Social Work: Thinking Beyond the Borders of the United States* (ed: Diane Drachman, and Ana Paulino) The Haworth Social Work Practice Press, an imprint of The Haworth Press, Inc., 2004, pp. 69-85. Single or multiple copies of this article are available for a fee from The Haworth Document Delivery Service [1-800-HAWORTH, 9:00 a.m. - 5:00 p.m. (EST). E-mail address: docdelivery@haworthpress.com].

Digital Object Identifier: 10.1300/J191v02n01_05

INTRODUCTION

The development of social work has been tied to the historical impact of migration and immigration from its inception. Both the Charity Organization and Settlement House movements focused their efforts on the influx of rural-to-urban and foreign-born migrants who came to reside in the "ghettoes" of United States cities. Concerns regarding poverty, deviance, family functioning and cultural assimilation motivated much of early social work theory and practice. The social work profession still deals with these concerns. How capable is social work in addressing the current needs of immigrants and refugees? This paper presents a discussion of Puerto Rican migration as a useful example for how social work practice with immigrants and refugees is related to political, economic, and cultural factors.

While there has been Puerto Rican migration to the mainland United States since the 1800s a sizable exodus began in the 1950s. Before World War II, Puerto Rican migration to the United States was minimal, but at the war's end there began a surge in Puerto Rican migration to the mainland resulting in a net migration of about 835,000 between 1940 and 1970. During that period, one out of every two Puerto Ricans born on the island migrated to the mainland making "Puerto Rico the site of one of the most massive emigration flows of this century" (Rivera-Batiz and Santiago, 1996, p. 43).

The demand for labor created by an expanding United States economy drew on contract labor from the island. This process was facilitated by close cooperation and planning between mainland employers, the United States government, and Puerto Rico's Department of Labor. After the most significant net outflow of Puerto Rican migrants in the 1950s and 1960s, outflows decreased dramatically in the 1970s, but escalated again between 1980 and 1990. In 1990, the Puerto Rican mainland population was 2.7 million. By 2000, this population increased to 3,406, 178, almost as much as the total population of Puerto Rico, which in that same year was 3,808,610. Currently Puerto Ricans are the second largest Latino group in the United States (US Bureau of the Census, 2001).

Since 1917, all Puerto Ricans, whether island- or mainland-born, are United States citizens. Physical proximity and relatively affordable transportation encourages Puerto Rican migration to the mainland United States. The fluctuations observed over the last four decades have had much to do with the changing economic, political, and cultural conditions on both the island and the mainland. Puerto Rican migration takes three forms: the "one-way migrants" who move permanently to the mainland; the "return migrants" who migrate to the mainland but after many years return to the island and reestablish residence; and the "circular migrants" who migrate back and forth between the island and the mainland spending substantial periods of residence in both places.

The phenomenon of Puerto Rican circular migration has been reported, discussed, investigated, and analyzed by journalists, policymakers, practitioners, and academic researchers (Melendez, Rodriguez, and Figueroa, 1991, p. 19). Although circular migration is not the dominant mode of migration among Puerto Ricans, "census-based measurements suggest that circular migration is a significant phenomenon among Puerto Ricans" (Rivera-Batiz and Santiago, 1996, p. 61). Approximately 130,335 Puerto Ricans were circular migrants in the 1980s, almost as many as the roughly 150,000 Puerto Ricans return migrants in that same period (Rivera-Batiz and Santiago, 1996). Generally, circular migration has been viewed in a negative light (Suro, 1998; Melendez, Rodriguez, and Figueroa, 1991; Tienda and Diaz, 1987). A number of problematic issues such as a lack of labor force commitment, disruptions in children's education, family disorganization, cultural disintegration, and resistance to cultural assimilation, have all been attributed to this pattern of migration (Rodriguez, 1998; Zentella, 1997; Melendez, Rodriguez, and Figueroa, 1991).

This article provides an analysis of Puerto Rican circular migration and contributes to the discussion of the more general theme of migration and immigration. The analysis emphasizes the conditions that instigate the departure of Puerto Rican migrants from both the island and the mainland, and discusses the implications of Puerto Rican circular migration for social work.

"NO SOY DE AQUI NI SOY DE ALLA"
("I'M NOT FROM HERE OR THERE")

Although Puerto Ricans exhibit a high rate of mobility similar to that of other ethnic and racial groups with significant numbers of immigrants, the barriers to the mobility of Puerto Ricans are substantively different from those of foreign-born immigrants (Rivera-Batiz and Santiago, 1996). Any comparison of Puerto Rican migration to that of foreign-born immigrants into the United States must recognize this. Yet, the research literature on immigration often treats Puerto Ricans similarly to foreign-born immigrants. Puerto Rico is a territory of the United States. Island-born Puerto Ricans, however, are considered distinct from those born in the mainland. These analytic compromises are the result of the political, economic, and cultural circumstances that place Puerto Rico "betwixt and between" strict definitions and categories.

The titles of a number of scholarly works testify to Puerto Rico's conflicted character: "Colonial Dilemma" (Melendez and Melendez, 1993) and "Island Paradox" (Rivera-Batiz and Santiago, 1996). Scholars and policy analysts have characterized the Puerto Rican population residing in the mainland United States in a similar manner. For example, Chavez (1991), in her analysis of Hispanic assimilation in the United States, devotes a chapter to "The Puerto Rican Exception." Puerto Rico has many tensions and contradictions. Sometimes referred to as a commonwealth, Puerto Rico is a territory of the United States, but administratively and culturally, it is a separate country governed under a political system: the "free associated state." The United States Census Bureau officially separates the mainland and island populations in their figures. Puerto Ricans on the island receive federal transfer payments. They serve in the United States military, but cannot vote in presidential elections. They have no voting representation in Congress, and pay no federal taxes.

Puerto Rico cannot enter into treaties and trade agreements with other foreign nations. The island's economy is treated as separate from the United States, and the island's government sends its own representatives to international diplomatic functions, such as inaugurations and funerals for heads-of-state, and to international competitions such as the Olympics and Miss Universe. Puerto Rico maintains a separate language and distinct traditions from the United States. Yet it is one of the most Americanized countries in the Caribbean and Latin America. The hybrid nature of Puerto Rico extends to the Puerto Rican population in the mainland. It is reflected in the processes of migration and transnationalism.

Puerto Rican Migration and Transnationalism

Transnationalism occurs when there are ongoing networks that facilitate exchanges between members of two or more nations. People, communication, and goods and services flow through these networks and migration tends to be continuous and bi-directional. Along with trade relations between the nations, the circulation of remittances (money that is sent back home, usually to relatives) also directly links their economies. Participants in these networks develop a sense of place and identity that incorporates cultural conditions at both ends of the network. In the process not only is identity altered, but the integrity of boundaries that determine nationality, citizenship, and culture are also changed.

Since 1898, the direct control of Puerto Rican economic and political development by United States policy has created and solidified powerful ideological and material links. The geographical proximity between the two countries encouraged their development. Militarily the two nations became closely linked, with Puerto Rico playing a central role in United States military strategic concerns in the Caribbean region. Military bases proliferated on the island. In addition to citizenship status, these cultural, economic, and military linkages have bred a sense of familiarity across the two cultures, and these linkages have facilitated Puerto Rican migration and transnationalism.

Puerto Rican Circular Migration

Puerto Rican out-migration has been massive in the last 60 years. Although establishing the proportions of one-way, return, and circular migrants is difficult, the use of census data makes this possible. "Net migration" represents the difference between in-migrants and out-migrants. According to Rivera-Batiz and Santiago, Puerto Rico's net migration peaked in 1950s, slowed in the 1960s, fell sharply in the 1970s, and surged again in the 1980s. The net outflow in the 1980s was 116,571 persons. Return migration peaked in the 1970s, although there were still close to 150,000 return migrants in the 1980s. Between 1980 and 1990, 316,173 persons entered Puerto Rico intending to reside there. Of these entrants to Puerto Rico, 50 percent were return migrants, 31.8 percent were those of Puerto Rican ancestry born outside the island, and 18.2 percent were foreign-born immigrants. There were 130,335 Puerto Rican circular migrants in the 1980s.

While the data from the 2000 census has not yet been fully compiled, released, and analyzed, there are strong indications that circular migration continues to be significant. For example, in the year 2000, of the estimated 270,220,360 residents in the United States, approximately 41, 359,248 resided in a different home the previous year. Of those residing in a different home the year before, 2,119,807 were abroad during that time. Of those living abroad the year before, 67,331 were residing in Puerto Rico (US Bureau of the Census, 2000). Puerto Rican circular migration remains an aspect of migration that has important implications for policy and practice, yet the phenomenon is not sufficiently explained by most theories and models of migration. Understanding the process of Puerto Rican circular migration would contribute to the literature on migration.

Theories of Migration

The "social fact" of migration is perhaps more inescapable than ever; "the emergence of international migration as a basic structural feature of nearly all industrialized countries testifies to the strength and coherence of the underlying forces" (Massey, Arango, Hugo, Kouaouci, Pellegrino, & Taylor, 1993, p. 432; 1994). As it has in the past, immigration policy has become a major international concern, and for many nations, immigration concerns have become a matter of national security. The expansion of mobility and communication in industrialized and post-industrialized society has accentuated these concerns.

As critical as these concerns are, the theoretical foundation for understanding international migration is not fully developed and "when it comes to international migration, popular thinking remains mired in nineteenth century concepts, models, and assumptions" (Massey et al., 1993, p. 432). There is no unified, coherent theory of international migration. Yet, "a full understanding of contemporary migratory processes will not be achieved by relying on the tools of one discipline alone, or by focusing on a single level of analysis" because "their complex, multifaceted nature requires a sophisticated theory that incorporates a variety of perspectives, levels, and assumptions" (Massey et al., 1993, p. 432). All theories of migration are based on different assumptions and explain some aspects of migration. Each model has some empirical support in the literature, and perhaps more important, there is insufficient evidence to reject any of the theories.

Puerto Rican migration is particularly representative of how difficult it is to analyze processes of international migration. The factors that determine the circumstances and choices of individuals, families, institutions, and communities, and who eventually becomes an out-, return-, or circular migrant are varied and complex. Theoretical and methodological sophistication are required to advance knowledge about migration. An essential part of this effort is to understand the dynamics between economic development and migration.

Political and Economic Development in Puerto Rico

After annexing the island, the initial focus of United States economic development policies for Puerto Rico was on land consolidation and the expansion of sugar cane production. By the late 1940s, after the collapse of the sugar economy, the United States turned its attention to expanding labor-intensive industrial production on the island. This industrialization plan, named Operation Bootstrap, set an important historical precedent. It relied on granting tax and tariff exemptions to United States corporations that invested in the island, and included substantial public investment in these private ventures. The abundant cheap labor on the island offered United States' companies another source of savings. At first industrial development was geared to such industries as heavy manufacturing and oil refining. Later it shifted to more capital-intensive industries like pharmaceuticals and other high technology enterprises. The basic formula of Operation Bootstrap is the dominant model for economic development today: reduce or eliminate trade restrictions and provide a source of low-cost labor to encourage foreign investment and stimulate exports. Because of the United States' policies Puerto Rico experienced one of the most rapid economic expansions ever. However, by the 1970s this economic progress stagnated.

Today, Puerto Rico is a mixed bag of economic outcomes (Rivera-Batiz and Santiago, 1996). In terms of GDP, exports, and imports it ranks highly compared to other Caribbean and Latin American countries. It also has a vibrant tourist industry. Conversely, Puerto Rico has unemployment and poverty rates that far surpass those of the mainland. Crime has reached almost epidemic proportions. The island relies heavily on public transfers from the United States, and the tax incentives to encourage investment are being minimized and gradually eliminated over time. This will likely curb future investment in the island by United States enterprises.

Operation Bootstrap also relied on encouraging out-migration to relieve pressures on the island stemming from its dense population. The United States government facilitated and encouraged United States' businesses to recruit labor from the island. Puerto Ricans were recruited for agricultural and manufacturing jobs located primarily in the Northeast region of the United States and Puerto Rican migrants flowed into the mainland. Although the manufacturing jobs that were the initial attraction have virtually disappeared, the migration flow continues. If the economic climate declines in Puerto Rico, migration to the mainland is likely to increase as some Puerto Ricans choose to seek their fortunes in the mainland.

Puerto Rican Well-Being in the Mainland

As an aggregate, the Puerto Rican population in the mainland United States has not had positive economic and social outcomes (Suro, 1998).

When compared to other Latino groups, non-Hispanic Whites, and Asian-Americans, Puerto Ricans generally rank lowest on such indicators as per capita and household income, unemployment and poverty rates, labor force participation, educational achievement, and rates of home ownership. Receipt of public assistance has been common in many Puerto Rican communities. The overall profile of Puerto Rican economic and social well-being closely resembles that of African-Americans and Native Americans (Massey, 1993). For decades, social problems such as crime, delinquency, and drug and alcohol abuse or addiction have plagued Puerto Rican communities in the mainland United States. These statistics have been used to substantiate the interpretations of a number of journalists, policy-makers, and scholars, whose explanations of Puerto Rican poverty and social disorganization have primarily stressed the behavioral and cultural deficiencies of Puerto Ricans rather than the social forces that shaped this experience.

The Puerto Rican experience in the mainland, particularly in New York City, is much too variegated to be understood through an aggregate profile. During the last fifty years, the mainland Puerto Rican population has experienced a split. Suro (1998) describes this process as an "extraordinary ethnic mitosis . . . roughly speaking, about half did well socially and economically. Upward economic mobility carried many to the suburbs and to the Sun Belt. The other half remained poor and sometimes got poorer, and the poor half was concentrated in city ghettos" (Suro, 1999, p. 154).

New York City became the hub of Puerto Rican migration activity and the largest and most long-standing Puerto Rican community in the mainland. Much of the current state of well being of Puerto Ricans in the mainland has to do with the fortunes of those who migrated to New York City, whose progress was impeded by urban renewal, gentrification, highway and public housing development, and even widespread arson. These developments literally destroyed what had been potentially thriving Puerto Rican neighborhoods. Suro notes, "By the late 1950s Puerto Ricans owned some four thousand businesses in New York, more than the black population, which was nearly twice as large" (Suro, 1998, p. 142). Displacement from these neighborhoods had a destructive effect on Puerto Rican community development:

> Because so many Puerto Ricans were displaced persons within the city, they never had a chance to develop the kind of enclave economy in which dollars are recycled through retail shops and other small businesses, gradually allowing a community to develop its

own base of entrepreneurial capital and credit worthiness. This, in turn, meant Puerto Ricans were all the more dependent on wage employment and welfare. They never had a chance to build the kind of kinship networks and local organizations so typical of Latin communities, including El Barrio at one time. Without that web of churches, informal associations, and small institutions, economic losses translated into social losses much more quickly. In addition, the displacements diluted the Puerto Ricans' political strength by scattering them through many electoral districts. (Suro, 1998, pp. 148-149)

These historical details are missing from many discussions about Puerto Rican well-being in the mainland.

Puerto Rican Migration and Global Political and Economic Development

The economic and social conditions in Puerto Rico and in the Puerto Rican communities in the mainland United States pose a difficult social welfare problem. Are the conditions in these two contexts related? What kinds of policies are needed to address these conditions? Should efforts be coordinated between the island and the mainland? What are the lessons to be learned with respect to policy formation from analyzing the relationship between migration and economic development?

At times policymakers have found it vexing to implement policies within the transnational context of Puerto Rican migration. For example, findings suggest that the effect of attempting to equalize wage rates by setting minimum wage policies in Puerto Rico to United States federal guidelines has been ineffectual in lessening out-migration from the island (Santiago, 1991). At least in part, this failure has resulted from "the mistaken notion that policies based on economic conditions in the United States could be successfully implemented under different economic circumstances in Puerto Rico" (Melendez, Rodriguez, and Figueroa, 1991, p. 20). This "indicates that policymakers need to reformulate their models of the existing economic interdependencies between Puerto Rico and the United States" (Melendez, Rodriguez, and Figueroa, 1991, p. 20). There is a wealth of empirical research supporting the case that economic factors such as wages and labor-markets are important determinants of Puerto Rican migration (Castillo-Freeman and

Freeman, 1992; Fleisher, 1963; Friedlander, 1965; Maldonado, 1976; Rivera-Batiz, 1989; Santiago, 1993; 1994).

What are the lessons to be learned from analyzing the relationship between migration and economic development? In terms of economic development, social well-being, and the experience of transnationalism, the case of Puerto Rico is particularly suited to analyzing how the political, economic, and cultural contexts that shape social conditions have been fundamentally altered in an era of "globalization."

According to Mato (1997) globalization is "a long-standing historical tendency toward the increasing interconnection of peoples, their cultures, and institutions" (Mato, 1997, p. 170). Keigher and Lowery (1998) utilize Midgeley's (1997) definition in their discussion of the health implications of globalization: "a process of global integration in which diverse peoples, economies, cultures, and political processes are increasingly subjected to international influences, and people are made aware of the role of these influences in their everyday lives" (Keigher and Lowery, 1998, p. 153). Wallerstein (1974, 1979, 1984) conceptualizes this process as a long-term, large-scale process of economic, historical and sociocultural change caused by the penetration of capitalist development into the non-capitalist zones of the world.

This process began as early as the 15th century with the European colonization of non-Western regions. It rapidly expanded after World War II and was institutionalized at the global level through the political and economic accords created at the United Nations Monetary and Financial Conference at Bretton Woods, New Hampshire in 1944. Ultimately, it evolved into a series of trade agreements initiated with the General Agreement on Tariffs and Trade (GATT) in 1947, and the formation of free trade zones such as the European Union, the Association of Southeast Asian Nations (ASEAN), and the North American Free Trade Agreement (NAFTA). The World Bank and International Monetary Fund (IMF) created in 1944 and 1945 respectively, and World Trade Organization (WTO) established in 1995, make up the current institutional structure of this global political economy.

Globalization, and its component urbanization and "modernization," created conditions where boundaries are more diffuse and nation states, organizations, identities are less defined. Mobility and flexibility have become increasingly necessary in the fluid state of globalization.

Hybrid forms of economy, polity, and culture have resulted from this process. The indeterminate nature of Puerto Rico is structural and cultural. Puerto Ricans are citizens of two countries who live in two cultures. Circular migration is a reflection of Puerto Rican indeterminacy and hybridity, and represents a functional adaptation to globalization.

Puerto Rican Circular Migration and Changing Labor Processes

Circular migration has been interpreted as "dysfunctional" (Tienda and Díaz, 1987; Suro, 1998). It may be that circular migration has acted as a "safety valve" for Puerto Ricans. When encountering difficult circumstances both on the island and in the mainland "the availability of ready escape routes meant that many Puerto Ricans never confronted the problems in either place, and they paid the price for their inconsistency" (Suro, 1998, p. 151).

From another vantage, it may be interpreted differently. Torres and Rodriguez (1991), recognizing "the everyday need and ability of Puerto Ricans to function within family networks or communities that are both bilingual and bicultural," referred to this circularity as "functional dual migration." Rather than reflecting "a commitment to neither place," it "implies a commitment to both cultures" (Torres and Rodriguez, 1991, p. 251).

Migration and alternative household formation are rational responses to globalization and its requisite mobility and flexibility. Globalization has placed "a steady pressure to break the link between household organization and territoriality . . . to detach more and more people from a commitment (physical, legal, and emotional) to a particular small unit of land" (Wallerstein, 1991, p. 109). The dissolution of boundaries at the cultural level meets the demands of globalization and contributes to the apparent disintegration of the Puerto Rican household. Puerto Rican migration and household formation are flexible, spatially and culturally.

The pressures of globalization have changed the nature of Puerto Rican households and social networks detaching them from their connections to territoriality and increasingly maximizing their income-pooling functions. When understood within this context Puerto Rican circular migration makes sense. Migration maximizes individual and household opportunities. Circular migration merely extends the flexibility demanded of capital and labor by prevailing economic circumstances.

Current political and economic conditions developed in response to declining corporate productivity and profitability within the United States' economy that became evident by the early 1970s. Among policy makers, this decline was considered the result of rigidity in: capital investments, systems of production, labor markets, and welfare-state government policy. The private sector responded through technological change and automation, the search for new product lines and market niches, geographic dispersal of production and distribution, mergers and corporate restructuring, and by accelerating the period for returns on investment capital (Harvey, 1990).

The logic of contemporary political and economic conditions (sometimes referred to as the "new" or "post-industrial" economy) "rests on flexibility with respect to labour processes, labour markets, products, and patterns of consumption" (Harvey, 1990, p.147). Flexibility encourages innovation, reduces costs, and generates increased profits. The expansion of the service economy, the relocation of United States' companies' productive facilities abroad, and the rise in part-time and temporary work are all outgrowths of this new economy. This new regime of production and accumulation of profits necessitated forms of political and social organization and regulation that have a hybrid character.

Puerto Rico offers a perfect example. Circular migration is a newer, more flexible mode of migration, and the free associated state established a newer and more flexible mode of political and economic regulation. Puerto Rican government is an administrative state without a sovereign nation. In many ways, Puerto Rico was an early experiment in, and an incubator for the prevailing global economy.

Social Work and Globalization

Understanding how the pressures of globalization have shaped Puerto Rican culture and migration must underlie any attempt to ameliorate the economic and social conditions in Puerto Rico and in the Puerto Rican communities in the mainland United States. The socioeconomic conditions in Puerto Rico, and those Puerto Ricans struggle with in the mainland, are best understood within the context of globalization. Generations of Puerto Ricans have struggled with high rates of poverty, unemployment, and underemployment, low wages, and low levels of educational attainment. Social problems such as crime, violence, and drug addiction at times appear insurmountable. Families are vulnerable to these instabilities. The high rate of female-headed households in the Puerto Rican population seems to testify to this fact.

In response to current political, economic, and cultural demands, new arrangements of family and community may be developing. This dynamic is even more critical given the centrality of the family as the basis for the Puerto Rican household. Rivera-Batiz and Santiago (1996) note that in "1990, 84 percent of all the households in Puerto Rico were families," while of all the households in the United States " . . . only 71 percent were also families" (p. 40). This contrast suggests that the "role of the family as a unit of social organization is on the average stronger in Puerto Rico than in the mainland United States" (p. 40). Puerto Rican families are organized around a political economy that encourages mobility yet challenges and may even undermine their natural support systems. In order to maximize the potential benefit of family and social support Puerto Rican households, families, and communities have responded flexibly.

There are other indicators of the alteration of family structure. For example, the divorce rate on the island. Puerto Rico "has by far the highest divorce rate in Latin America and the Caribbean, with the exception of Cuba" (Rivera-Batiz and Santiago, 1996, p. 39). Family size has changed. The effects of family planning policies and socioeconomic factors have had an impact on fertility rates on the island. Over the last 60 years, Puerto Rican women have increased levels of educational attainment and they have become increasingly urbanized; two factors associated with declining fertility (Rivera-Batiz and Santiago, 1996). Clearly, the changing patterns in Puerto Rican family formation are not merely behavioral manifestations of moral frailties; like the process of circular migration, they are by-products of political economic development.

The social work practitioner should recognize that Puerto Rican families and communities present a distinct migration pattern that sets them apart from the typical immigrant experience. Political, economic, and cultural hybridity have created a unique set of linguistic and other cultural barriers to service provision in Puerto Rican communities. For example, because of Puerto Rican citizenship status, geographic proximity, and familiarity with United States culture, the acculturation experience (the level of cultural "assimilation" or incorporation of an individual to a "foreign" or receiving society) for Puerto Ricans is very different from most other immigrant populations. Also significant is the disruption caused by Puerto Rican mobility to the continuity of service provision. This has implications in that many models of service provision for immigrants and refugees adopt a linear stage approach to migration (Drachman, 1992), which while useful models for interpreting the typical immigrant experience, are less applicable to Puerto Ricans.

CONCLUSION

Whatever the domain of social work practitioners, whether in child welfare, juvenile justice, mental and physical health, or community and policy practice, social work must be able to serve individuals, families and households, and communities living in an era of globalization.

Advocacy and policy efforts to assist immigrants and refugees will be more effective if the profession begins to design strategies and tactics that take into account the current global political economy and how it determines public policy. For example, social work should be able to contribute more concretely to policy-making related not only to social policy and community economic development, but also to public policy at the global level such as international trade agreements. A human rights perspective would accomplish this (Reichert, 2001; Witkin, 1998). Social work should have an increased emphasis on human rights: civil, political, social, cultural, and perhaps most importantly economic. The full integration of a human rights perspective into social work would further efforts to develop, and advocate for, policies that might effectively address the needs of individuals, families, and communities in the current political, economic, and cultural environment. Research and education are important institutional resources in developing the capabilities of social work practice with immigrant and refugee populations. Social work research must focus more empirical attention on migration. An increased emphasis on international social work is a useful way to further these efforts. The profession must be equally active as a local, global, and transnational agent.

The Implications of "9/11"

Shortly after the completion of the original draft of this paper, the events of September 11, 2001 transpired. The editors have requested that the authors in this volume briefly discuss how the incidents on and after September 11, 2001 have affected the population discussed in the paper. Obviously, because New York City is home to the largest Puerto Rican community in the mainland US, the effects were immediate within the Puerto Rican population.

For many Puerto Ricans the "post-9/11" environment has re-opened old wounds and complicated the political relationship between the island and the United States. Although Puerto Ricans are not immigrants they are often treated as "foreigners" because of cultural differences. As one of the trends in the "post-9/11" environment has been an increasing atmosphere of deep mistrust, suspicion, and at times, blatant repression of the foreign-born, Puerto Ricans have become likely targets of this xenophobia.

In addition, there is a long-standing tension between the United States and those on the island and in the mainland who have advocated for Puerto Rican independence. At times in the past, this tension has manifested itself in acts of violence that were perpetrated by some elements in the independence movement. In the 1950s, Puerto Rican Nationalists attempted to assassinate President Truman and attacked the chambers of Congress shooting several representatives in the assault. In the 1980s, there was a well-publicized attack by an independence group Los Macheteros on an armored car in West Hartford, Connecticut. Most recently, there has been a popular coalition of various organizations conducting a civil disobedience campaign calling for the removal of the United States naval base on the island of Vieques (an offshore municipality of Puerto Rico). Before "9/11," the movement had accomplished much towards achieving that goal. Although the campaign was eventually successful, the process was somewhat derailed because of "post-9/11" militarization and the greater likelihood of the public perceiving this movement as "un-American."

Lastly, the economic impact has affected both the island and Puerto Ricans in mainland United States. The repercussions of "9/11" aggravated what had already been a fragile economic climate in the United States. For Puerto Ricans, this may have disastrous results. Many Puerto Ricans, both in New York City and the island, are employed in the service sector of the labor market such as food services and retail sales. This sector has been one of the hardest hit by the recent economic downturn. The downturn has also been detrimental to the tourist and travel industry, a primary aspect of the island economy. These circumstances could dampen the prospects of many Puerto Ricans. The consequences may be dire for a population that already is rife with unemployment and poverty. The exact nature of these potential changes are subject to speculation, but it is not hard to imagine that the political and economic aftermath of "9/11" will likely affect the migration decisions of many Puerto Ricans and will probably modulate the rate of circular migration.

REFERENCES

Castillo-Freeman, A., & Freeman, R. (1992). When the minimum wage really bites: The effect of the U.S. level minimum on Puerto Rico. In G. Borjas & R. Freeman (Eds.), *Immigration and the workforce* (pp. 177-211). Chicago: University of Chicago Press.

Chavez, L. (1991). *Out of the barrio: Toward a new politics of Hispanic assimilation.* New York Basic Books.

Drachman, D. (1992) A stage-of-migration framework for service to immigrant populations. *Social Work, 37* (1): 68-72.

Fleisher, B. (1963). Some economic aspects of Puerto Rican migration to the United States. *Review of Economics and Statistics.*

Friedlander, S. (1965). *Labor migration and economic growth.* Cambridge, MA.: MIT Press.

Giddens, A. (2000). *Runaway world: How globalisation is reshaping our lives.* London: Routledge.

Hannerz, U. (1996). *Transnational connections: Culture, people, places.* New York: Routledge.

Harvey, D. (1990). *The condition of postmodernity.* Cambridge, MA: Blackwell.

Katz, M. B. (1989). *The undeserving poor: From the war on poverty to the war on welfare.* New York: Pantheon Books.

Keigher, S.M. & Lowery, C.T. (1998). The sickening implications of globalization. *Health & Social Work, 23,* 2, 153-158.

Lewis, O. (1966). *La vida: A Puerto Rican family in the culture of poverty–San Juan and New York.* New York: Random House.

López, A. (1987). *Doña Licha's island: Modern colonialism in Puerto Rico.* Boston: South End Press.

Maldonado, R. (1976, September). Why Puerto Ricans migrated to the United States, 1947-1973? *Monthly Labor Review.*

Massey, D., Arango, J., Hugo, G., Kouaouci, A., Pellegrino, A. & Taylor, J. E. (1993). Theories of international migration: An integration and appraisal. *Population and Development Review, 19,* 431-466.

Massey, D., Arango, J., Hugo, G., Kouaouci, A., Pellegrino, A. & Taylor, J. E. (1994). An evaluation of international migration theory: The North American case. *Population and Development Review, 20*: 699-751.

Melendez, E. & Melendez, E. (Eds.). (1993) *Colonial dilemma: A critical perspective on contemporary Puerto Rico.* Boston, MA: South End Press.

Melendez, E., Rodriguez, C., & Figueroa, J. (1991). Hispanics in the labor force: An introduction to issues and approaches. In E. Melendez, C. Rodriguez & J. Barry Figueroa (Eds.), *Hispanics in the labor force: Issues and policies* (pp.1-24). New York: Plenum.

Midgeley, J. (1997). Social welfare in global context. Thousand Oaks, CA: Sage Publications.

Offe, C. (1984). *Contradictions of the welfare state.* Cambridge, MA.: The MIT Press.

Reichert, E. (2001). Placing human rights at the center of the social work profession. *The Journal of Intergroup Relations, 28,* 1, 43-50.

Rivera-Batiz, F. (1989, October). The Characteristics of recent Puerto Ricans migrants: Some further evidence. *Migration World.*

Rivera-Batiz, F., & Santiago, C. (1996). *Island paradox: Puerto Rico in the 1990s.* New York: Russell Sage Foundation.

Rodriguez, C. E. (1998). Puerto Rico and the circular migration thesis. *Journal of Hispanic Policy, 3,* 5-9.

Santiago, C. (1991). Wage policies, employment, and Puerto Rican migration. In E. Melendez, C. Rodriguez & J. Barry Figueroa (Eds.), *Hispanics in the labor force: Issues and policies* (pp. 225- 246). New York: Plenum.

Santiago, C. (1993). The migratory impact of minimum wage legislation: Puerto Rico 1970-1987. *International Migration Review, 27*, 4, 772-95.

Santiago, C. (1994). The changing role of migration in Puerto Rican economic development: Perspective from the past and look to the future. In C. Torre, H. Rodríguez & W. Burgos (Eds.), *The commuter nation: Perspectives on Puerto Rican migration (pp. 171-186). Río Piedras, P.R: University of Puerto Rico Press.*

Suro, R. (1998). *Strangers among us: Latino lives in a changing America.* New York: Vintage.

Tienda, M., & Diaz, W. (1987, August 28). Puerto Rican circular migration. *New York Times.*

Torre, C.A., Rodriguez, H., & Burgos, W. (Eds.). (1994). *The commuter nation: Perspectives on Puerto Rican migration.* Río Piedras, P.R.: University of Puerto Rico Press.

Torres, A. & Rodriguez, C.E. (1991). Latino research and policy: The Puerto Rican case. In E. Melendez, C. Rodriguez & J. Barry Figueroa (Eds.), *Hispanics in the labor force: Issues and policies* (pp. 247-264). New York: Plenum.

US Bureau of the Census. (2000). *Census 2000 supplementary summery tables: Residence 1 year ago for the population 1 year and over.* Washington, DC: U.S. Government Printing Office.

US Bureau of the Census. (2001). *Census 2000 brief: The Hispanic population.* Washington, DC: U.S. Government Printing Office.

Vásquez Calzada, J. (1988). *La población de Puerto Rico y su trayectoria histórica.* Río Piedras, P.R: Raga Printing.

Wallerstein, I. (1991). Household structures and the labour-force formation in the capitalist world-economy. In E. Balibar & I. Wallerstein (Eds.), *Race, nation, class: Ambiguous identities* (pp. 107-112). London: Verso.

Waters, M. (1995). *Globalization.* London: Routledge.

Witkin, S. (1998). Human rights and social work. *Social Work, 43*(3): 197-201.

Zentella, A.C. (1997). Returned migration, language, and identity: Puerto Rican bilinguals in dos worlds/two mundos. In Darder, A., Torres, R.D., & Gutiérrez (Eds.), *Latinos and education: A critical reader* (pp. 302-318). New York: Routledge.

On the Age Against the Poor: Dominican Migration to the United States

Ramona Hernández

SUMMARY. This article focuses on Dominican migration to the United States (U.S.) after 1965. Dominicans left their homeland pressured by economic needs, the desire to improve their lives, and encouraged by a de facto immigration policy that facilitated their exodus. Once in the U.S., most Dominicans encounter an economy that increasingly demands skills and levels of schooling they do not possess. Rather than a prosperous life, in the new land, Dominicans face high unemployment levels and an alarming state of poverty. Paradoxically, while the needs of Dominicans continue to be unmet in the new society, the social policies and the conditions that push them out of their country remain in effect. On its part, the U.S. has responded by adopting a number of immigration laws to control the entrance of unwanted and unneeded job-seekers. As a result, the number of Dominicans coming to the U.S. has begun to decline as the number of Dominicans deported to the Dominican Republic has increased. In the end, poor Dominicans are pushed back and forth by both societies whose immigration policies mask their unwillingness to respond to the needs of the group. The article also discusses the impact on the Dominican community of 9/11 and the crashing of the AA flight 587, on November 12, 2001. *[Article copies available for a fee from The Haworth Document Delivery Service: 1-800-HAWORTH. E-mail address: <docdelivery@haworthpress.com> Website: <http://www.HaworthPress. com> © 2004 by The Haworth Press, Inc. All rights reserved.]*

Ramona Hernández, PhD, is Director, Dominican Studies Institute, and Associate Professor, Sociology Department, City University of New York.

[Haworth co-indexing entry note]: "On the Age Against the Poor: Dominican Migration to the United States." Hernández, Ramona. Co-published simultaneously in *Journal of Immigrant & Refugee Services* (The Haworth Social Work Practice Press, an imprint of The Haworth Press) Vol. 2, No. 1/2, 2004, pp. 87-107; and: *Immigrants and Social Work: Thinking Beyond the Borders of the United States* (ed: Diane Drachman, and Ana Paulino) The Haworth Social Work Practice Press, an imprint of The Haworth Press, Inc., 2004, pp. 87-107. Single or multiple copies of this article are available for a fee from The Haworth Document Delivery Service [1-800-HAWORTH, 9:00 a.m. - 5:00 p.m. (EST). E-mail address: docdelivery@haworthpress.com].

http://www.haworthpress.com/web/JIRS
Digital Object Identifier: 10.1300/J191v02n01_06

KEYWORDS. Dominican Republic, Dominican migration, immigration, migration, policy

EMIGRATION FROM THE DOMINICAN REPUBLIC

Massive emigration from the Dominican Republic began in 1962 after the death of dictator Rafael Leónidas Trujillo, who ruled the country tyrannically from 1930 to 1961. During the dictatorship, international migration was severely restricted and only a few Dominicans, particularly diplomats and well-to-do people who were known to favor the government, were granted visas. Two reasons have been advanced to explain Trujillo's restrictive emigration policies: first, by limiting emigration the dictatorial regime prevented dissatisfied Dominicans from mounting outside any political campaign against the government; second, constraining emigration contributed to the growth of the population, a policy emphasized by the government as the basis for economic development.

During Trujillo's regime, the Dominican Republic embarked on a development strategy based primarily on the modernization of the agricultural sector, the expansion of agricultural production, and the development of an industrial complex. That model was promoted under the conviction that the Dominican Republic lacked enough people to satisfy the needs of the emerging productive market, and therefore, emigration was severely restricted and child births were systematically encouraged. During Trujillo, production was organized under the assumption that Dominicans were needed as workers and consumers to advance the economic development of the country. Consequently, any unabsorbed contingent of workers at any given moment was perceived as a necessary surplus and was prevented from emigrating.

After Trujillo's assassination, the number of Dominicans admitted under permanent status (with "Green Card") to the United States increased to 10,683 from the 1962 number of 4,603. The number of people coming to the U.S. continued to increase progressively, as witnessed in the annual number of Dominicans who left their homeland between 1962 and 1991. Between 1962 and 1972 the annual mean of Dominican migrants was 11,445. This number increased to over 16,000 during the 1970s and to over 30,000 during the 1980s. In 1991 and 1992 the number of Dominicans admitted reached over 40,000 each year (Statistical Year Book of Immigration and Naturalization Service, 1991). The following section will look at those who come from the Dominican Republic.

A PROFILE OF THE MIGRANTS

A careful examination of the occupational backgrounds of most Dominican migrants coming to the United States would indicate that most Dominicans come from the underprivileged sectors of the Dominican Republic and that they possess low educational attainment (see Table 1). According to Immigration and Naturalization Service (INS) data, most Dominicans admitted to the U.S. were predominantly manual and bluecollar workers, including domestic servants. In 1970 only 6.6% of Dominicans admitted to the U.S. reported being professional, technical, and kindred workers and 24.5% of them reported being operatives. In 1972 only 8% of Dominicans admitted held occupations as professional, technical, and kindred workers, but 29% of them were classified as operative workers. In 1977, the pattern continued, showing a 6% of Dominicans admitted as professional, technical, and kindred workers, and a 19.9% of them admitted as operative workers (INS Annual Reports 1970; 1972; 1977). Table 2 indicates that during the 1980s the number of Dominican males classified as operators, fabricators, and laborers is 4.5 times higher than the number admitted as professional, specialist, and technician.

During the 1970s, arguably 1 out of every 4 Dominicans migrating to the United States was likely to be a blue-collar worker, specifically, an operative, and 3 in every 50 had a professional or technical career. During the same decade, less than 1 out of every 2 Dominicans was likely to have an occupation at the time of migrating to the United States. During the 1980s, the pattern slightly changed since many more Dominicans, particularly males, reported to have an occupation before departure. Although blue-collar workers continued to dominate the migratory flow by a very large margin, that decade featured more professional and technical workers migrating than during the 1970s. The data reflect that during the 1980s more than 1 out of every 2 Dominican males was likely to have an occupation before migration, while less than 1 out of every 2 women was likely to have an occupation. Similarly, 2 out of every 25 Dominican males were likely to have a professional or technical skill, while approximately 9 out of every 25 were likely to be an operative. Out of every 14 women admitted, 1 reported to have a professional or technical career and 1 out of every 8 women was likely to be an operative worker.

The increase in the number of professional and technical workers migrating from the Dominican Republic during the 1980s, as compared to the 1970s, corresponded to the progressive deterioration of the public

TABLE 1. The Educational Status of the Population in New York City 1990, 1996 (Persons 25 years of age or older in %)

Population Group	Percentage of the Population Completing:							
	Less than High School		High School		Some College		College or More	
	1990	1996	1990	1996	1990	1996	1990	1996
Dominican	52.3	54.7	20.4	25.0	19.3	16.3	8.0	4.0
NYC	20.8	24.1	24.8	31.5	24.5	17.6	29.9	26.8
Non-HW	11.7	12.0	23.2	29.8	23.5	18.0	41.6	40.2
Non-HB	24.9	25.5	29.9	39.7	29.6	22.0	15.6	12.8
Hispanic	40.4	48.4	25.6	28.4	23.1	15.2	10.9	8.0

Source: Hernández, Ramona, and Francisco Rivera-Batiz 1997.

TABLE 2. Percent Distribution of Dominican Male and Female Immigrants 16 to 64 Years Old with an Occupation in New York City 1982-1989

	Male	Female
Total with an Occupation	23,699	16,604
Professional, Specialty, and Technical	8.0	7.0
Executive, Admin, and Managerial	6.8	2.3
Sales	5.3	2.9
Admin. Support	6.2	10.3
Precision, Prod., Craft, and Repair	18.3	15.8
Operator, Fabricator, and Laborer	36.6	12.9
Farming, Forestry, and Fishing	8.4	0.2
Service	10.3	48.6

Source: Department of City Planning 1992: 83; 86.

services, the drastic fall of the value of the *peso*, and the loss of stable and well-paid jobs in the sending society. The 1980s was the decade of the intervention of the International Monetary Fund and its austerity plan. By 1991, the purchasing power of the minimum wage reflected half the value it had in the 1970s. And salary readjustment in the large companies of the modern sector brought these salaries down to 60% of their value in the 1970s. During the 1980s, many members of the middle class sectors could not escape the negative effects of the economic changes occurring in the country. This time, they too were heavily impacted.

If, during the 1970s, the middle class in particular benefited from the expatriation of surplus laborers and the direct transferring of resources from the poor and less privileged sectors, the economic restructuring of the 1980s provoked the dislocation of a more diverse group, directly affecting many members of the middle class sectors and pushing them to seek the same solution constantly sought by the less privileged groups.

EXPLAINING THE EXODUS

Massive migration from the Dominican Republic developed in response to the socioeconomic policies implemented in the Dominican Republic after 1966. Upon assuming the direction of the Dominican State in 1966, the Balaguer government tackled two principal concerns: economic development and political stability. Economically, the government implemented a model that eased the entrance of United States investment and tended to emphasize industrial production, commercial trade and finance. Politically, Balaguer put in place a reign of terror that virtually dismembered the opposition through frequent incarcerations, assassinations, and the expatriation of political dissidents. During Balaguer's first 12-year regime, the Dominican Republic would be characterized by dichotomous tendencies. On the one hand, there was unprecedented economic growth, via the expansion of industrial production and the business sectors. Between 1970 and 1974 industrial production grew at an annual rate of 120% (Duarte and Corten 1982). On the other hand, there were growing unemployment levels provoked by the intensification of industrial capital, an inadequate policy of job-growth, and the internal mobilizations of uprooted people in search of jobs from the countryside to the city (see Table 3).

From 1970 to 1974, the Dominican Republic experienced the highest economic growth rate of any Latin American country, with an average return profit in net gains of over 54% in the industrial sector. Between 1970 and 1977, the capital invested in the food industry increased from DR$130.9 million to DR$196.8 million, and in the intermediary industry, from RD$31.2 million to DR$70.5 million (Vicens 1982). At the same time, during the same years the country had an official unemployment rate of over 20%. Over half of the working people were underemployed. The bottom fifth of the population with the lowest income experienced an extraordinary loss, reflecting a fall of over half its income. And 75% of the people did not consume the number of calories and nutrients required to maintain an adequate diet.

TABLE 3. Unemployment Rates in the Dominican Republic

(% of Labor Force)	
Year	(%)
1970	24.1
1973*	20.0
1978*	24.4
1979*	19.3
1980	22.2
1981	20.7
1982	21.3
1983	22.1
1984	24.2
1985	27.2
1986	28.7
1987	25.0
1988	20.8
1989	19.6
1990	19.7
1991	26.6
1993	37.6
1996	37.6

Sources: for 1970-1979, Ceara Hatton 1990b: 60. For 1980-1991, Ceara Hatton and Croes Hernández 1993:18. For 1993 and 1996, Ramirez, 1999:8.

Neither the administrations of the Partido Revolucionario Dominicano, which ruled the country from 1978 to 1986, nor that of the returning Balaguer in the period 1986-90, generated any improvement in the lives of most people at home. During the 1980's, or "the lost decade," in the words of Dominican economist Bernardo Vega, most workers who needed to work for a living suffered. Many were displaced from the process of production by an economy that systematically introduced technology into production and increasingly depended on a labor force that possessed formal schooling and training. By 1984, 40.8% of the children under 5 years of age were malnourished, and the number of families below the poverty level had doubled, rising to 47%, and increasing again by 1989 to 56% (Santana and Rathe 1993:189).

In spite of the economic booms of the last years of the 1990's, poverty and unemployment rates in the Dominican Republic have remained consistently high. In 1993 the Oficina Nacional de Planificación concluded that 60% of the Dominican homes were poor. Four years later, the same official institution reported that 56% of Dominican homes were poor and that almost one in five lived in a state of indigence. In 1993, the unemployment rate in the Dominican Republic was 26.2% and by 1996, it had increased to 37.6% (Ramírez 1999:8). In a study conducted by the International Labor Organization it was found that the informal economy provided 50% of all urban jobs in the Dominican Republic in 1997. The same study found that among all the seven countries studied, the Dominican Republic, with a GNP annual average growth of 4.1%, experienced the highest economic growth since 1994 but the lowest growth of the labor force during the same years (Del Cid and Tacsan Chen 1998:12).

But what explains the migration of Dominicans specifically to the United States? The implementation of the new economic model and social stabilization in the Dominican Republic was assumed with two objectives in mind, the reduction of birth and the annihilation of political dissidence. Both goals entailed the complicity of the States from the Dominican Republic and the United States.

AN EVIL ALLIANCE: CAPITAL AND THE STATES

President Joaquín Balaguer took office on June 1, 1966 and by April 23, 1968, his government had already approved a new investment law, Law No. 299 of Industrial and Incentives Protection, which henceforward served as the basis for capitalist accumulation in the country. After intense negotiations, the new industrial law was finally approved. Law 299 offered a number of incentives which facilitated industrial expansion, ranging from the removal or the reduction of tariffs, to the provision of infrastructure for the development of industrial complexes. The new law also tried to prevent direct competition among foreign and national capitalists by channeling foreign investments to new areas of production which native capitalists could not develop. The promulgation of this law institutionalized a tripartite model of accumulation in the country constituted by the government, the private sector, and international capital. Each one depended and leaned on the other to sustain the new established social order. This collaboration would be fundamental for the development of a migratory movement to the United States.

Balaguer's political consolidation and control of the country was required if the economic plan was to succeed. Consolidation involved a pacification of the country through political repression, killings, and in-carcerations. The modernization of the army and the national police forces, with assistance from the Pentagon and the CIA, provided the nec-essary infrastructure to ruthlessly impose order by the sword in the country, as may be gathered from the fact that Balaguer's first two terms in government left a toll of over 3,000 people killed (Moya Pons 1995). The pacification also included opening the doors to expel undesirable voices that attacked the regime, and who represented an immediate threat to the new social order. Through an unwritten and undeclared agreement between both the U.S. and the Dominican governments, po-litical dissidents were granted visas by the American consulate and were directly dispatched to the United States. But the magnitude of the exodus experienced by Dominican society after 1966 suggests that the opening was used not only to eliminate unwanted political dissidents, but also other Dominicans, perhaps those for whom the system had no use.

The opening of the door for Dominicans to leave did not need an offi-cial promulgation from the government. It simply became a tacit agree-ment among the players. Dominicans would apply for a passport and the government would simply grant it. Contrary to Trujillo's time, now vir-tually any one who wanted a passport could have it. Commenting on this, Frank Canelo points out that while in 1959, 19,631 people applied for a passport and only 1,805 got one, in 1969, every petition out of the 63,595 that applied received approval (1982:42). The granting of pass-ports concretized the opening of the door and, through the opening of the door, emigration was tacitly encouraged on the part of the ruling structure in the Dominican Republic.

Although the Dominican government did not stipulate or even sug-gest that the emigration of people was needed to reduce population pres-sure, it is now clear that at the time the size of the population was a matter of concern. If the mobilization of people, unofficially encour-aged, was managed in such a way that any one could simply believe that migration was the result of an individual decision rather than the result of an intended and decided political strategy on the part of the Domini-can power structure, this was not the case for population control. A drastic control of population growth was firmly and clearly imposed by the Dominican State. Shortly after Balaguer took office in 1966, a Na-tional Family Planning Program was instituted. The program was inte-grated by the Asociación Dominicana Pro-Bienestar de la Familia (PRO FAMILIA), a U.S. agency established in 1966 and financed by the American International Development Agency, and by the Consejo Nacional de Población y Familia, an official government agency created in 1968 to complement the efforts of PROFAMILIA.

Statistics indicate that the implementation of family planning (FP) in the Dominican Republic has been successful. After the 1960's, the fertility rate fell sharply in the country. While in 1955, for instance, the average fertility among Dominican women was close to 8 children per woman, in the 1955-95 period, this number had been reduced to 3.2, placing the Dominican Republic among the four countries with the lowest fertility rates in Latin America. During the quinquennium 2020-2025, it is expected fertility rate to further drop to a projected 2.6 or 1.9 children per woman, depending on whether one assumes a conservative or a more reductionist approach (*Las proyecciones de población en la República Dominicana*: 7). For the past five decades or so, major population changes in the Dominican Republic have been determined primarily by fertility rates. Consequently, the sharp decline in fertility among women has caused population growth rate to decline from an average annual growth rate of 3.5% in the 70s, to 2.3% in the 1980s, to a projected 1.6% between 1990 and 2010 (*The Economist* 1990:17; 22).

The implementation of FP in the Dominican Republic was not a conjunctural decision on the part of the U.S. Nor was it the result of an awareness about population growth on the part of the Dominican people as Bernardo Vega has suggested (Vega 1990:260). On the contrary. FP in the Dominican Republic responded to a long-term U.S. foreign policy on population control, particularly directed to areas recipient of U.S. capital investments. FP was first approved for Puerto Rico under the idea that there was a population excess in that island. It was believed that population pressure in the island was the cause of extreme poverty and high unemployment rates, which were an obstacle to socioeconomic progress. By 1968, while industrial production was still booming in Puerto Rico, "35 percent of the women between twenty and forty nine years of age had been sterilized–a proportion several times larger than the closest comparable figure for any other country" (History and Migration Task Force 1979:132).

FP was disseminated throughout the Latin American region under the auspices of the Agency for International Development which from 1968 to 1972 had a designated operating capital of 100 million dollars. By 1986, there were 4,000 FP workers in the Dominican Republic charged with the task of disseminating a new ideology among people. People, particularly the poor and women, were told that their poverty had to do with their procreation of children, and that they needed to curtail their procreation patterns. The perception of poverty as an individual choice, rather than as a social issue, legitimized the state of inequality in the Dominican society and exonerated the state, the power structure, and the privileged social sectors from distributing and sharing society's wealth. As it was played out in the Dominican Republic, the adoption of FP by Dominican women was not the result of an individual, or a woman's choice. All seems to indicate that in this country FP was an imposed social policy to reduce population pressures.

II

The collaboration of the U.S. and the Dominican government in the implementation of FP in the Dominican Republic clearly suggests that both perceived population growth in this country as a problem and were interested in controlling it. The cooperation of the U.S. with the Dominican government in the development of the Dominican emigration, on the other hand, was the result of a conjuncture in which both agents were guided by different goals. Emigration from the Dominican Republic to the United States was encouraged by U.S. representatives as a short-term measure to eliminate an immediate problem. They saw the deportation of revolutionaries who challenged the government of Balaguer and the established new social order "as temporary." The Dominican power structure, on the contrary, perceived the emigration of people, not just as a temporary strategy by which political discontent could be eliminated. Rather they saw it as a long-term policy through which dissidence as well as excess labor could be easily eliminated.

The emigration of Dominicans to the U.S. was not formally discussed with the U.S. government during Balaguer's administrations. Vega emphasized that from 1961 to 1982 basically two issues dominated the discussions between the U.S. and the Dominican governments: the sugar quota and the amount of aid for the Dominican Republic (Vega 1990: 82). Although, as noted by Vega, there was no discussion on the part of both governments on the issue of emigration, a door had conveniently opened for Dominicans to emigrate to the United States.

EXPLAINING THE RECEIVING SOCIETY

According to the U.S. census, in 1990 there were 511,297 Dominicans living in the United States, and over 65% of them were residing in the state of New York alone. By 2000, the number of Dominicans in the

U.S. had increased to 1,041,910 and in New York City to 554,638. In 1990, New York City in particular accounted for over 93% of those Dominicans who were living in the New York State area. As indicated in Table 4, from 1980 to 1990 the Dominican population of the city increased from 125,380 to 332,713 to become the ethnic group with the largest growth in the city for that period. Their remarkable numerical gain was the result of a constant and growing immigration influx, combined to high fertility rates among Dominican women, particularly in New York City. In 2000, 53.2% of all Dominicans residing in the United States lived in New York City. The massive arrival of Dominicans occurred at a time when New York City was undergoing a socioeconomic restructuring in the labor market. This transformation would have a remarkable impact on the need for and value of labor as well as in the creation of jobs.

The restructuring of the city involved a transformation from an economy based predominantly on industrial production to one based on services. As a result of this change, today New York City is commonly classified as a post-industrial city. Scholars generally agree that some time during the 1950s the large manufacturing sector which had characterized the economic life of the city began to shrink. The shrinking process manifested itself in the disappearance of hundreds of thousands of manufacturing jobs, particularly in the garment industry, the largest area of industrial production in the city. From 1969 to 1985, for instance, the city lost 465,000 manufacturing jobs (Drennan 1991:29). The restructuring process dislocated productive jobs directly as well as a whole variety of other jobs that were tangentially connected to the manufacturing sector. Entire industrial headquarters moved out, and with them their employment opportunities. From 1969 to 1989, for instance, employment in wholesale trade declined from 309,000 to 229,000, and in trucking and warehousing from 41,000 to 26,000 (Drennan 1991:32). But overall, the decline in employment occurred primarily among blue-collar and unskilled workers who suffered from 1970 to 1986 the loss of 510,000 jobs in fields that required less than twelve years of education (Kasarda 1990:247).

The arrival of Dominicans in the United States coincided also with the massive entrance into the country of other immigrants who were attracted to the same job market. Coming mostly from Asia, Latin America, and the Caribbean regions, immigrants tended to concentrate in large metropolitan cities, where they expected to find entry-level jobs at the bottom of the market. During the 1970s and 1980s, along with thousands of Dominicans, thousands of other immigrants, particularly His-

TABLE 4. The Dominican Population of New York City, by Borough

New York City Borough	Number 1980	1990	% of Total 1990	Number 2000	% of Total 2000
Manhattan	62,660	136,696	41.1	185,808	33.5
The Bronx	17,640	87,261	26.2	181,450	32.7
Brooklyn	21,140	55,301	16.6	95,267	17.2
Queens	23,780	52,309	15.7	89,567	16.1
Staten Island	160	1,146	0.4	2,545	0.5
Total	125,380	332,713	100.0	554,637	100.0

Source: Hernández, Ramona, Francisco Rivera-Batiz, and Roberto Agodini 1995.

panics and West Indians, settled in New York City. Yet, the city had experienced an economic transformation that radically changed the needs of the labor market. Native low-and-unskilled-blue collar workers, particularly from ethnic minorities, could not withstand the high unemployment levels and declining industrial demand. They began to abandon the city massively, while large numbers of immigrants, expecting to find jobs, began to enter. By 1990, despite the large immigration influx, New York City still had almost one million people less than it had in 1960. The declining demand for blue-collar and unskilled workers and the increasing influx of immigrants would have serious negative repercussions for all city workers searching for unskilled jobs. The combination of a declining demand and an enlarging supply of workers of similar skills would generate competition among job-seekers, native and foreign born, and their easy substitution by employers. Such a situation would negatively impact the lives of Dominican families.

In effect, as reflected on Tables 5-7, Dominicans residing in New York City had the highest levels of poverty and unemployment rates for 19980, 1990 and 1996 when compared to other large racial or ethnic groups. The persistent high rate of poverty among Dominicans is a direct result of a number of socioeconomic variables including low earnings, high incidence of female-headed families with low earnings, employment instability due to structural economic transformation and the loss of blue-collar and low-and-unskilled jobs, particularly in the manufacturing sector, spatial segregation in low-growth job areas, such as the inner city versus the suburbs, and low educational attainment in a school-knowledge based society.

"Passing Back the Bucket"

The United States has closed its door. The immigration policies adopt ed in the United States since the mid 1980s have begun to have their effects on the number of people coming from the Dominican Republic. As a matter of fact, in 1996, the number of Dominicans admitted to the United States actually began to decline. In 1998, only 20,387 Dominicans were admitted to the U.S. This figure represents less than half of the Dominicans admitted seven years before. Besides limiting the number of those admitted, other measures were put in place to reduce unwanted immigrants.

In 1980, we witnessed a shift in the U.S. government's thinking about Third World immigrants. The "benign neglect" approach ceased

TABLE 5. Poverty Rate in New York City, 1980, 1990, 1996

Population Groups	Poverty Rate in %		
	1980	1990	1996
Dominican Population	36.0	36.6	45.7
New York City Average	18.0	17.2	23.8
Non-Hispanic Whites	8.7	8.2	11.2
Non-Hispanic Blacks	28.3	22.9	33.1
Hispanic Population Overall	35.0	31.4	37.2

Sources: for 1980 and 1990: Hernández, Ramona, Francisco Rivera-Batiz, and Roberto Agodini 1995; for 1996: Hernández, Ramona and Francisco Rivera-Batiz 1997.

TABLE 6. Unemployment Rates in New York City 1980, 1990, 1996
(Persons 16 years of age or older)

Population Group	Unemployment Rate in %					
	Male			Female		
	1980	1990	1996	1980	1990	1996
Dominican	14.3	15.1	18.9	9.5	18.4	18.6
New York City	7.0	8.7	10.3	6.6	8.1	9.0
Non-Hispanic White	5.0	5.5	7.1	5.1	4.9	5.9
Non-Hispanic Black	13.1	14.3	18.0	9.9	10.9	13.6
Hispanic Overall	14.0	12.4	12.6	12.2	13.6	12.0

Source: for 1980 and 1990: Hernández, Ramona, Francisco Rivera-Batiz, and Roberto Agodini 1995; for 1996: Hernández, Ramona and Francisco Rivera-Batiz 1997.

TABLE 7. Family Type and Poverty Rate, 1990 (in %)

Population Groups	Married-Couple Rate	Poverty Headed	Female-Rate	Poverty
Dominicans	38.1	20.8	40.2	58.5
Puerto Ricans	33.8	14.5	36.0	57.9
Colombians	46.9	9.4	20.3	27.5
Ecuadorians	53.8	12.2	12.9	39.6

Source: Hernández, Ramona 2002.

to exist as the dominant response to the entrance of unneeded immigrants. Legislative efforts began to be introduced which proposed a firm attitude towards unwanted job-seekers coming in. As the decade progressed, various immigration laws were approved. It became increasingly clear that the State no longer wished to maintain a passive or even merely discursive attitude toward the immigrant flows. With the Immigration Reform and Control Act of 1986, which specifically targeted and penalized employers who hired foreign-born workers who did not have proper work-authorization, the State initiated a new modality for regulating and controlling the entrance of migrants. Firm, aggressive, and often punitive measures now became part of immigration legislation.

Benign indifference gave way to an aggressive offensive policy against immigrants coming from the Third World, particularly from Latin America and Asia. Legislation was supported by a mass of federal funds. Sophisticated devices such as infrared scopes and eye glasses, contrived for use at night to inspect the border with Mexico, which had become an international bridge facilitating the influx of people from Latin America, the Caribbean, and Asia. At the border, to keep intruders out, tall cement walls were erected. In addition, the INS employed electrified fences, ferocious and well-trained dogs, special police troops, and other paraphernalia to contain the flow of undocumented immigrants. In the Tucson area, for instance, 1,380 agents were posted in May 2000. Authorities claimed that an overwhelming amount of uninvited guests were coming in and that they were catching approximately 900 of them per day. The decision was to secure the area well by posting three agents per mile along the border between the town of Douglas and the Naco station, an area which agents believed had been targeted by incoming immigrants (Zaragoza 2000). In effect, in the town of Douglas, a citizen who has decided to take action on his own to help authorities deal with the unwelcome influxes, is offering tourists a new kind of sport-adventure, a man-hunt. The citizen in question is " . . . offering winter vacationers a radical departure from mainstream entertainment. He is inviting winter visitors to come to the Southwest, set their recreational vehicles on ranch property, and help capture elusive illegal entrants as they make their nocturnal trek across the Sonoran Desert" (Zaragoza 2000).

While until then the new policies had only targeted undocumented migrants, in the middle of the 1990s, the focus expanded to include documented ones as a pervasive anti-immigration climate took hold of the land. Spokespersons against documented immigration raised their voices. Suddenly, policy-makers became concerned about the need for an urgent action concerning the nation's surplus unskilled foreign workers. Propositions of curtailing immigration flourished among government representatives from the states of Florida, California, Texas, and Louisiana. In June 1992, Senator Robert C. Byrd shared this incident with his peers in the Senate: "I pick up the telephone and call the local garage. I can't understand the person on the other side of the line. I am not sure he can understand me. They're all over the place, and they can't speak English. Do we want more of this?" (Sontag 1992:E5). The answer to his question came in the form of two new laws enacted during 1997: the Anti-Terrorist Act and the Welfare Reform Act. Both legislative acts have been perceived as anti-immigrant. In the process, the anti-immigration climate at the governmental level has succeeded in winning over representative voices from civil society. A national survey on the issue of immigration conducted by Gallup in 1994 revealed that 65% of the American people wanted legal immigration curtailed.

The pervasive anti-immigration wave has reached a peak. Voices adversarial to the influx of Third World immigrants are being heard loud and clear in every corner of this country. Washington no longer desires to send an unclear message regarding immigration: unequipped immigrant job-seekers are no longer welcome. Employers have not mounted any opposition. Unwanted job-seekers, their children included, must be ready to deal with an inimical ambience. Up to December of 1999, more than 177,000 people had been deported to their countries of origin. Among those deported, some had criminal records indicating minor offenses, such as smoking marijuana at a younger age or evading to pay a fare for public transportation. Others deported, however, simply lacked proper documentation. The INS has set annual targets for deporting undocumented and criminals. By 1999, however, INS managed to surpass its own set quota. In 1999, the quota was put at 120,000, which represented a 3% increase from the previous year. Yet, in November of the same year, the number of deportees already reached 57,000 more than the accorded quota for the year (a 142% increase). In the specific case of the Dominican Republic, Table 8 reflects that the number of those sent back home for various reasons has steadily increased since 1965. While 633 Dominicans were deported between 1965 and 1969, the number of Dominicans deported during the 1995-1998 period increased to 8,757. For now, however, the answer of the sending societies to Washington's new immigration policies continues to be formulated according to these countries' needs.

Deportation laws are severe. Deportees, particularly criminals, are likely to be permanently barred from entering legally to the United States. While the United States continues to maintain an aggressive policy deporting Dominican immigrants left and right, the effects of deportation are devastating among Dominican families both in the US as well as in the Dominican Republic. It is likely that the removal of a head of a household will not only affect the socioeconomic standing of this person's household here in the US, but it will also put an end to this person's ability to send remittances to family members in the Dominican Republic. Social workers in community based organizations located within Dominican communities in New York City argue that deportations break families apart, often leaving children in single households and unable to see one of their parents. Social workers also argue that a good number of children of Dominican ancestry who come from sin-

TABLE 8. Dominicans Deported to Country of Birth

Year	Number Deported
1965-1969	633
1970-1974	612
1975-1979	909
1980-1984*	914
1985-1989**	1,198
1990-1994	4,544
1995-1998***	8,757

*Does not include data for the following years: 1980, 1981, and 1982.
**Does not include data for 1985 and 1988.
***Latest date available.
Source: *INS Annual Reports*, 1965 to 1998.

gle-female-headed families and whose mothers have been deported to the Dominican Republic, end up in adoptive homes/institutions, and are forced to lose contact with the only parent they have known.

TRAGEDY HITS DOMINICAN PEOPLE HARD

The Impact of September 11th

On September 11th, 2001, two airplanes en-route to New York City were abruptly taken by terrorists and crashed against the World Trade Center (WTC). As of February 21st, 2003, 2,743 persons had been reported as victims of the WTC attack. Among the reported deaths, 263 were of Hispanic ancestry and 27 of them had been born in the Dominican Republic (Hernandez & Rivera-Batiz, 2003). Like many other New Yorkers, Dominicans were doubly affected by the WTC tragedy. Some Dominicans lost members of their families, people who were known to them, or people for whom they worked. Yet, the attack on the WTC had a more pervasive disturbing effect in the life of the New York City Dominican community as a whole. The destruction of the WTC affected Dominicans both from an economic and psychological point of view. Dominicans were affected by the economic crisis directly created by high unemployment levels among them and among all other workers in the city. With unemployment, the multiplying effect of their salary was lost. Unemployed Dominicans had to limit their buying power, and this created a domino effect in the economic life of the Dominican community: it impinged in the life of the *bodegas*, general stores, Dominican street vendors, and home-babysitters, among others.

The attack also created a sense of fear among Dominicans who felt vulnerable in social places. Governmental authorities, through the power of the media, propagated the belief/idea that another terrorist attack was imminent and that no one was safe. People were asked to be vigilant, watchful, suspicious, and ready to denounce to the authorities any action/package they thought they could not explain/recognize. As many New Yorkers, Dominicans were influenced by the ugly view and the smell of burning smoke left on the site where the two majestic buildings were located. As all New Yorkers, they were also constantly reminded about death and the number of innocent people who were killed during the tragic event of September 11th, 2001.

The Impact of American Airline Flight 587

Two months and one day exactly after the WTC attack, Dominicans underwent another tragedy. On November 12th, 2001, an American Airline plane, flight 587, crashed in Rockaway, Queens, a few minutes after taking off from John F. Kennedy International Airport. The plane exploded in the air shortly after taking off, killing instantly 265 people, 260 on board the plane, 5 people on the ground. The plane was en-route to Santo Domingo, the capital city of the Dominican Republic. As Table 9 indicates, among the deaths, 187 had been born in the Dominican Republic and the majority of those who died resided in New York City, particularly in the Bronx and Manhattan. In addition, among the deceased, 218 were of Hispanic ancestry and 118 of them were women. Among those who died, 119 of them were between 30 and 54 years of age and only 34 of them were senior citizens (between 65 and 85 years of age).

The crashing of the AA flight 587 has been classified as the disaster that has taken the second highest number of lives in the history of New York City. It is also the second highest death toll in the US aviation history.

Without a doubt, the loss of lives in the plane crash affected the economic well-being of Dominicans here as well as in the Dominican Republic. Most of the Dominicans who died were within active economic-ages and their deaths directly affected the families they supported in both places. Needless to say that as with the tragic event of 9/11, the well-being of the entire Dominican community was affected by the loss of productive lives.

But the loss of lives also brought pain and a sense of fear for the Dominican community. Dominicans discussed the tragedy everywhere: in schools, in radio programs, in the corners, in the *bodegas*, and in the intimacy of their homes with their families and friends. The news about the crashing of the flight also permeated the Dominican Republic: they too were fearful and unable to explain what had happened. To make matters worse, no one, either from the American Airline side or The National Safety Board, could explain why or what caused the plane to crash. Of course, the inability to explain the reasons behind the incident made many Dominicans doubtful and skeptical about American Airline's capacity to prevent another plane from crashing and killing Dominicans in the future.

Two years have passed since the event involving flight 587. In examining the news covering the event, published on November 12th, 2002 in New York City papers, one finds that many Dominicans have not

TABLE 9. Birthplace and Residence of Decedents

Birthplace	Number
Dominican Republic	187
USA	58
Puerto Rico	1
All Other Places	15
Residence	
New York City	191
Manhattan	60
Bronx	65
Brooklyn	32
Queens	33
Staten Island	1
New York State	
Outside NYC	25
United States	
Outside NYS	30
Rest of the World	19
Total	**265**

Source: *Summary of Vital Statistics 200, The City of New York.* Bureau of Vital Statistics, New York City Department of Health and Mental Hygiene, March 2003.

been able to put the matter to rest and that many of them continue to speak about feeling fearful and having a sense of hopelessness. This is true particularly among family members of the victims. Family members interviewed by newspaper reporters complained about the City's lack of response to their request of creating a memorial on the site where the plane crashed. In addition, opposition to erecting the memorial on the site also emanates from residents of Belle Harbor, the neighborhood where the airplane crashed. Yet, many Dominicans, including community leaders, believe that a memorial remembering the victims should be erected on the spot where many Dominicans unexpectedly succumbed to death.

Although no study has yet been conducted measuring the strength of the Dominican community in responding to both devastating events—the 9/11 and the AA flight 587–one can empirically see that the community has survived and continues to try to move forward. As a people, Dominicans are no exception to the rule: during trying times involving social tragedies, people tend to pull together and find courage to deal with the adversity that affects them. The fact that Dominicans have not forgotten the plane crash and the pain they went through, does not mean that they, as a community, will be paralyzed and dedicate their time to re-living the nightmare they experienced on November 12th, 2001 at 9:16 AM. The Dominican community is a migrant community that is pushed by the spirit of economic progress and social stability that brought them here in the first place. The Dominican community is also motivated by the need to see their children succeed in the new land where they were born.

REFERENCES

Bureau of Vital Statistics, March, 2003. New York City Department of Health & Mental Hygiene.

Ceara Hatton, Miguel. 1990. *Crecimiento económico y acumulación de capital: Consideraciones teóricas y empíricas en la República Dominicana.* Santo Domingo: Universidad Iberoamericana (UNIBE).

Ceara Hatton, Miguel and Edwin C. Hernández. 1993. *El gasto público social de la República Dominicana en la década de los ochentas.* Santo Domingo: Centro de Investigación Económica y Fondo de las Naciones Unidas para la Infancia.

Del Cid, Miguel and Rodolfo Tacsan Chen. 1999. *Fuerza Laboral, Ingresos y Poder Adquisitivo de los salarios en Centroamerica, Panama, y Republica Dominicana: 1998. Organizacion Internacional del Trabajo.* Costa Rica: LIL, S.A.

Department of City Planning. 1991. *Annual Report on Social Indicators.* New York City: Department of City Planning.

_____ 1992. *The Newest New Yorkers: An Analysis of Immigration into New York City During the 1980s.* New York City: Department of City Planning.

Drennan, Matthew. 1991. "The Decline and Rice of the New York Economy." In *Dual City: Restructuring New York.* Edited by John Mollonkop and Manuel Castells, 25-41. New York City: Russell Sage Foundation.

Duarte, Isis and Andre Corten, 1982. "Proceso de proletarizacion de mujeres: Las trabajadoras de industria de ensamblaje en Republica Dominicana." Typescript.

Frank Canelo, J. 1982. Dónde, por qué, de qué, y cómo viven los dominicanos en el extranjero: un informe sociológico sobre la e/inmigración dominicana, 1961-62. Santo Domingo: Alfa y Omega.

Hernández, Ramona. 2002. *The Mobility of Workers Under Advanced Capitalism: Dominican Migration to the United States.* New York: Columbia University Press.

Hernández, Ramona, Francisco Rivera-Batiz and Roberto Agodini. 1995. *Dominican New Yorkers: A Socio-Economic Profile.* New York City: CUNY Dominican Studies Institute at the City College of New York.

Hernández, Ramona and Francisco Rivera-Batiz. 1997. *Dominican New Yorkers: A Socio-Economic Profile*. New York City: CUNY Dominican Studies Institute at the City College of New York.

Hernández, Ramona and Francisco Rivera-Batiz. 2003. *Dominican New Yorkers: A Socio-Economic Profile*. New York City: CUNY Dominican Studies Institute at the City College of New York.

History and Migration Task Force, Centro de Estudios Puertorriqueños. 1979. *Labor Migration Under Capitalism: The Puerto Rican Experience*. New York: Monthly Review Press.

Immigration and Naturalization Service 1960-1991. Statistical Yearbook of the Immigration and Naturalization Service. Washington, DC: G.P.O.

Kasarda, D. John. 1990. Structural Factors Affecting the Location and Timing of Urban Underclass Growth. *Urban Geography* II:234-64.

Las Proyecciones de poblacion en la Republica Dominicana 1990-2005. Santo Domingo: Centro de Estudios Sociales y Demograficos and Oficina Nacional de Planificacion Nacional.

Moya Pons, Frank. 1995. *The Dominican Republic: A National History*. New York: Hispaniola Books.

_____. 1993. *La emigración dominicana hacia el exterior*. Santo Domingo: Instituto de Estudios de Población y Desarrollo.

_____. 1993. *La fuerza de trabajo en la República Dominicana*. Santo Domingo: Instituto de Estudios de Población y Desarrollo.

Ramirez, Nelson (1999). "Un pais a la media: Distorciones en la medicion de la pobreza y el desempleo en la Republica Dominicana." Santo Domingo. Centro de Estudios Sociales y Demograficos (CESDEM).

Santana, Isidoro and Magdalena Rathe. 1993. *Reforma social: Una agenda para combatir la pobreza*. Santo Domingo: Editora Alfa y Omega.

Sontag, Deborah. 1992. "Calls to Restrict Immigration Come from Many Quarters." *The New York Times* (December 13):E5.

The Economist. 1990. *Book of Vital World Statistics: A Portrait of Everything Significant in the World Today*. New York: Times Books, a division of Random House, Inc.

Vega, Bernardo. 1990. *En la década perdida*. Santo Domingo: Fundación Cultural Dominicana.

Vicens, Lucas. 1982. *Crisis económica 1978-1982*. Santo Domingo: Editora Alfa y Omega.

Zaragoza, Xavier. 2000. "Borane Is Not Amused With > Ranch Watch = Flyer." *The Daily Dispatch* (April 20):1A.

Return Migration: An Overview

Charles Guzzetta

SUMMARY. Immigration to the United States (U.S.) is made for many different reasons, which may be economic, political, or social or any combination of them, and subsequent reverse migration may occur for any of the same reasons. Discussion of immigration and the variety of circumstances attendant to it are wide-ranging, but usually such discussions rely on figures related to migration into the country and overlook, either purposefully or accidentally the fact that return migration has always been a significant movement in this country. This article raises the issue of limited data gathering by the U.S. on reverse migration despite the sizeable amount and quite reliable demographic information on arrivals. Discussions of social services for immigrants, therefore, cannot be considered complete or even competent if they do not include careful consideration of and attention to return migration. *[Article copies available for a fee from The Haworth Document Delivery Service: 1-800-HAWORTH. E-mail address: <docdelivery@haworthpress.com> Website: <http://www. HaworthPress.com> © 2004 by The Haworth Press, Inc. All rights reserved.]*

KEYWORDS. Return migration, reverse migration, migration, immigration

---

Charles Guzzetta is Professor, Hunter College School of Social Work, City University of New York.

[Haworth co-indexing entry note]: "Return Migration: An Overview." Guzzetta, Charles. Co-published simultaneously in *Journal of Immigrant & Refugee Services* (The Haworth Social Work Practice Press, an imprint of The Haworth Press) Vol. 2, No. 1/2, 2004, pp. 109-117; and: *Immigrants and Social Work: Thinking Beyond the Borders of the United States* (ed: Diane Drachman, and Ana Paulino) The Haworth Social Work Practice Press, an imprint of The Haworth Press, Inc., 2004, pp. 109-117. Single or multiple copies of this article are available for a fee from The Haworth Document Delivery Service [1-800-HAWORTH, 9:00 a.m. - 5:00 p.m. (EST). E-mail address: docdelivery@haworthpress.com].

Digital Object Identifier: 10.1300/J191v02n01_07

DEMOGRAPHIC BRIEF

Studies of immigrant populations tend to view immigration as a one-way stream. Scholarly research on the topic is abundant, varied and impressive, often examining the distribution and impact (both social and economic) of immigration trends. Social service providers typically rely upon demographic impact studies to propose policies and services involving immigrant populations. However, in almost all proposals for services for immigrants, one fundamental phenomenon is quite consistently ignored; namely, that a significant proportion of all immigrants who enter a country return to their home countries. The discussions of immigration, whether by proponents of services for immigrants or opponents of immigration, tend to use only incoming numbers, not "net migration"; that is, the figures for those who came minus the figures for those who returned. As Smith and Edmonston (1997: 36) put it: "There have been emigrants as long as there have been immigrants." They estimate that between 35% and 45% of all immigrants leave, either to go back home or to travel to a third country. The special circumstances of their sojourn in the United States and their special needs in returning to their native homes qualify as an important area of activity for social workers. Immigration is a much more complex phenomenon than it once seemed to be.

The perception among social workers, of immigration as a one-way movement of people is seen in the policy statement of the International Federation of Social Workers (IFSW). With no supporting documentation, the statement claims that people usually migrate "for work" (2000). Throughout the policy statement, the burden of adaptation and service provision placed on the receiving country; return migration is not mentioned at all. As a practical matter, information about immigrants who return is essential for government and private agency policymakers. For example, the Social Security Administration must calculate projections on applications, eligibility, and scope of retirement benefits. But, as Smith and Edmonston (1997: 39) observe, while demographic data on incoming migrants are quite reliable, data on outmigration are "particularly scarce and elusive." The Social Security Administration suggests that a third of all immigrants subsequently emigrate (Smith and Edmonston 1997: 40, footnote #17), while the Immigration and Naturalization Service , which does not collect data on emigration, estimates the rate of return migration to fall between 20% and 25% (Bouvier 1992: 34). In the absence of hard data on emigration, rough estimates have to be used with all the policy perils inevitably related to using imprecise information.

RETURNEES:
A UNITED STATES HISTORICAL PHENOMENON

The phenomenon of reverse migration or return migration (to note some of the terms used) has become a major area of scholarly study only during the last few years, during which the research has ballooned, although as Gans (1999) has pointed out, there still are many "holes" in the research. One reason this field of study was overlooked for so long is that hard data seemed difficult to determine, a problem that continues to dog the work of researchers in the field. The importance of such data seems to have been a long-standing subject of debate in government, given the uneven record of government policy on the matter. Isbister (1996: 3) flatly declared that the U.S. government "keeps no statistics on emigration," although *immigrants* are carefully counted. It is held that emigrants "tend to be shadowy and elusive, whereas immigrants are highly visible . . . " (Dashevsky et al. 1992). Apparently, this was not always the case. In 1819, a law required all ships to list passengers by citizenship; an "official record of emigrants began in 1907" (Historical Abstracts 1961:49), counting as "emigrants" those "aliens who have resided in the United States for a year or longer and who are leaving. . . . " The government record of "returnees" began in 1908, according to Foerster (1919), but it was based on records of disembarking ship passengers at European ports and were unreliable even in that simple accounting. Not only have reliable data not been systematically collected, there is not even agreement about which data are relevant for collection. One authority in the field argued that "there is much terminological sloppiness in the . . . literature" (King 1986: 3), giving consistency of opinions about emigration a highly elusive quality even though it is the bedrock of understanding and prediction.

Three decades ago, one researcher concluded that "a meaningful number" of immigrants return to their homelands. Although without precise information about the rate of return, he estimated that it was such that "the net gain in population due to immigration in the United States was something between fifty and eighty percent of the accepted figures" (Axelrod 1972: 46-47).

Although return migration as an area of research interest has grown rapidly only during the past two or three decades, it has a long history.

Over eighty years ago, Foerster (1919) reported that statistics kept by the U.S. on immigrants listed them as either "permanent" or "temporary." During the time of his review, 1876 to 1903, the "temporary" groups always outnumbered the "permanent" group. One of the seminal pieces of work was published a mere thirty years ago. In it, Bovenkerk (1974) sought to provide a sense of system to the almost random approaches he found in the research. In his work, he was seeking only to name and explain immigration, not to quantify any of it. Quantification is one area that has continued to elude scholars, partly because of the lack of agreement on terminology.

As previously stated, return migration is not a movement of recent origin. It has been happening for as long as people have been migrating, but it was made significantly more practical (as was the original migration) by the development of steamship transportation which provided relatively cheap, fast and safe passage across wide expanses of water by the middle of the 19th century (Caroli: 1990). Reverse migration, as well as other kinds of long-distance migration, accelerated again with the introduction of cheap air travel via the Boeing 747 planes in the mid-20th century. However, even when travel was both prohibitively expensive and extremely hazardous, people left North America in great numbers to "go back home." Wyman (1994:4) claims that in New England during first half of the 1600s, " . . . those returning to England outnumbered those going to America . . . ," an assertion supported by Caroli (1990: 24), who gave the striking example that of Harvard's first class of nine graduates, seven returned to England.

As already noted, the return home from the United States of immigrants during the great boom in immigration between 1880 and 1920 also reached high levels, although the rate of return seems to have varied for different countries. Examining the return flow of immigrants during the period from 1908 to 1923, Wyman (1993: 11) found the rate of return generally high, but much higher for some countries than for others, ranging from 40% returning to Poland and 60% to southern Italy, to about 52% returning to Russia and 66% to Slovakia.

UNDERSTANDING THE PHENOMENON
OF REVERSE MIGRATION

Part of the problem in understanding the phenomenon of reverse migration may flow from the widespread assumption that immigrants intend to stay in the countries to which they go, including the United

States. Perhaps, *especially* the United States! A certain justifiable pride in the United States as the "land of opportunity" may support this assumption, but available data do not. The assumption possibly relates to the likelihood that many of the writers on the topic themselves are descended from immigrants whose stories of the "old country" are colored by the misery, poverty and oppression that led to the original family exodus. However, it has been observed that it is incorrect even to assume that most of the immigrants originally *intended* to stay. As study of the field progressed, it became increasingly clear that the one-way assumption was invalid. In fact, King (2000) flatly claims that most immigrants intend to return to their homelands when they come to this country (as noted earlier by Foerster).

RETURNEES: AN INTERNATIONAL PHENOMENON

Reverse immigration is not limited to the United States; it is seen wherever there is immigration, world-wide. For example, Greenwood and Young (1997:5) recently reported that in Canada, "a large portion of [the] immigrant population subsequently departs. . . ." Australia seems to have similar figures; "about 20 to 30 percent of the English-speaking immigrants" to that country later leave (Beenstock 1996: 950). According to Kurthen (1995:935), Germany has been subject to "extensive immigration and outmigration . . . since the earliest historical records. . . ." Even more striking are the figures from Israel, where about 40% of the "young, single immigrants" from North America return "within three years" of their arrival (Beenstock 1996:950).

SOME REASONS WHY IMMIGRANTS RETURN

Both the reasons for and the rate of return migration seem to have been influenced by a variety of factors. Bovenkerk (1974) and later, following Bovenkerk, King (1986) proposed four "intentions" for migration, in relation to migration outcome. The scheme included: (1) migration intended to be permanent and, in fact, permanent; (2) migration intended to be permanent but with return migration; (3) migration intended to be temporary and with return migration; and (4) migration intended to be temporary, but becoming permanent. These four types of "intentions and outcomes" cover a variety of immigrant intentions and an equal variety of outcomes, half of which are not the migrants' intended outcomes. This disparity raises the question of why return migration takes place, and why it takes place with far greater frequency than is generally acknowledged. Two reasons for return migration seem to predominate: because they fail or because they succeed. Obviously, this seeming paradox encompasses many different possible specific reasons. Rogers (1984) presented a list of eight reasons which she found in her research. They included: changes in the home country which made return either feasible or profitable or both; awareness of being needed in the home country, either by family or for patriotic reasons; changes in the receiving country which made staying there no longer feasible; or disappointment over inability to achieve the goals that had induced the original migration. In his studies of Italian immigrants, Cerase (1967, 1974) found reasons which are consistent with the Rogers list; he noted that both economic success and economic failure in America, plus attachment to traditional Italian values influenced decisions to return. King (2000) found that the reasons for returning fell into four broad categories: social, economic, political, and family.

There is little disagreement that the major reason for migration to the United States has almost always been economic, and economic reasons figure prominently among those given for return migration. Many immigrants learn skills or techniques (especially in agriculture) that they take back home, but Kritz and her associates (1992) found that many of them became "reimmigrants" because of better opportunities to have what they consider a good life here. King (2000) further claimed that the longer the immigrants were away, and the farther from their home country they had migrated, the less likely they were to return. Moreover, he argued that the more closely the culture of the receiving country resembled that of the sending country, the more likely the return migration. Although he did not provide statistical data to support that assertion, it would seem to be reflected in the high return rates among the countries of the British Commonwealth of nations, for example. King, Straehen and Mortimer (1983) also stated that high return rates revealed a pattern comprising three major types: between countries approximately alike in development; from developing countries back to industrial countries; and sojourners in industrial countries back to less developed homelands. Suro (1996) identified other factors that seemed to influence the likelihood and rate of return migration. He found that single immigrants who married locals and started families were less likely to return to their home countries, while immigrants who married partners from the home country were more likely to return. This view seems consistent with the observation of Bovenkerk (1974: 23) that "a certain amount of integration in the receiving country is a necessary condition for success and as integration proceeds, the chance of return diminishes."

IMPLICATIONS

Immigration to the United States is made for many different reasons, which may be economic, political, or social or any combination of them, and subsequent reverse migration may occur for any of the same reasons. Discussion of immigration and the variety of circumstances attendant to it are wide-ranging, but usually such discussions rely only on figures related to migration into the country and overlook, either purposefully or accidentally the fact that return migration always has been a significant movement in this country. The rate of reverse migration fluctuates with economic conditions (both in the sending country and the receiving country), and in relation to other factors, such as political conditions (again, in both countries), culture, and social/family considerations.

There is general agreement that in case of a major downturn in the U.S. economy, remittances would decline, return migration would be likely to increase sharply and this would have profound consequences for the sending countries (Russell 1986), with ripple effects in the United States. In any case, the phenomenon of return migration is regrettably ignored in discussions of immigration and its impact on the U.S. society and its economy.

Return immigrants who go home may also face daunting challenges. Wiest (2000), an anthropologist, pointed out that a major factor faced by returnees is the stress of changed social mobility. We simply do not know how returnees relate to the people who stayed in the home country, nor how the returnees are received by them. An unavoidable conclusion from Wiest's observation is that social services cannot focus exclusively on immigrants who are assumed to be coming to the U.S. to stay, since a major portion of them will not do so, but need to address the sorts of problems migrants will face upon going back. Finally, policies and programs based upon the largely erroneous assumption that all immigrants intend to stay here overlook another powerful influence on immigrants: the policies and programs of their native countries to attract them back. Since the 1970s, Gnosh (2000:131) reports, all the major European countries "have developed policies and programmes to assist return." Included are help with transportation costs, with housing, employment, social security benefits, and other inducements.

Effective work with immigrants, as Martin (2001) cogently argues, requires a solid grasp of complex world politics, recognition of changing concepts of nationality and familiarity with the growing range of national and international organizations that provide services to migrants. In short, discussion about social services for immigrants cannot be considered complete or even competent if they do not include careful consideration of and attention to return migration.

REFERENCES

Axelrod, B. (1972). Historical studies of emigration from the United States. *International Migration Review* 6:1 (Spring), pp. 32-49.

Beenstock, M. (1996). Failure to absorb: Remigration by immigrants into Israel. *International Migration Review* 30:4 (Winter), pp. 950-978.

Bouvier, L. (1992). *Peaceful Invasion.* New York: University Press of America.

Bovenkirk, F. (1974). *Sociology of Return Migration: A Bibliographic Essay.* The Hague: Martinus Nijhoff.

Caroli, B. (1990). *Immigrants Who Returned Home.* New York: Chelsea House.

Cerase, F. (1974). Expectations and reality: A case study of return migration from the United States to southern Italy. *International Migration Review* 8:2 (Summer), pp. 245-262.

Cerase, F. (1967). A study of Italian migrants returning from the U.S.A. *International Migration Review* 1:3 (Summer), pp. 57-74.

Dashevsky, A., J. DeAmicus, B. Lazerwitz & E. Tabony (1992). *Americans Abroad: A Comparative Study of Emigrants from the United States.* New York: Plenum Press.

Foerster, R. (1919). *Italian Immigration of Our Times.* New York: Russell & Russell.

Gans, H. (1999). Filling some holes. *American Behavioral Scientist* 42:9 (June/July), pp. 1302-1313.

Gnosh, B. (2000). Return migration: Reshaping policy approaches. In B. Gnosh (Ed.), *Return Migration: Journey of Hope or Despair.* Geneva: International Organization of Migration.

Greenwood, M. & P. Young (1997). Geographically indirect immigration to Canada: Description and analysis. *International Migration Review* 31:1 (Spring), pp. 51-71.

Historical Statistics of the United States (1961). Washington: United States Government Printing Office.

Ibister, J. (1996). *Immigration Debate.* West Hartford: Kumarian Press.

International Federation of Social Workers (1998). *International Policy on Refugees.* IFSW Policy Papers (Publications, updated, 2000).

King, R. (2000). Generalization from the history of return migration. In B. Gnosh (Ed.), *Return Migration: Journey of Hope or Despair,* pp. 7-55. Geneva: International Organization of Migration.

King, R., A. Strachen & J. Mortimer (1983). *Return Migration: A Review of the Literature.* Oxford: Oxford Polytechnic.

King, R. (Ed.) (1986). *Return Migration and Regional Economic Problems*. London: Croom Helm.

Kritz, M., L. Lim & H. Zlotnik (Eds.) *International Migration Systems*. Oxford: Clarendon Press.

Kurthen, H. (1995). Germany at the crossroads: National identity and the challenge of immigration. *International Migration Review* 29:4 (Winter), pp. 915-938.

Martin, S. (2001). Forced migration and professionalism. *International Migration Review* 35:1 (Spring), pp. 226-243.

Rogers, R. (1984). Return migration in comparative perspective. In D. Kubat (Ed.), *The Politics of Return*. Proceedings from the European Conference on International Migration Return. New York: Center for Migration Studies.

Russell, S. (1986). Remittances from international migration: A review in perspective. *World Development* 14:6, pp. 677-696.

Smith, J. & B. Edmonston (Eds.) (1997). *The New Americans*. Washington: National Academy Press.

Suro, R. (1996). *Watching America's Door*. New York: Twentieth Century Fund Press.

Wiest, R. (2000). Anthropological perspectives on return migration: A critical commentary. In B. Gnosh (Ed.), *Return Migration: Journey of Hope or Despair*, 167-196. Geneva: International Organization of Migration.

Wyman, M. (1993). *Round Trip to America: The Immigrants Return to Europe, 1880-1930*. Ithaca: Cornell University Press.

Mexican Immigrants:
"Would You Sacrifice Your Life for a Job?"

Maria Zuniga

SUMMARY. Social Work's history is embedded in this profession's service and commitment to immigrant populations. This new century presents itself with a new mixture of immigrants who come to United States (U.S.) shores seeking a better life. The challenge to social workers is to be well-versed in social policy, human behavior, and practice realms related to serving these immigrants. Schools of social work must insure that curriculum reflects the needs and situations of this new mix of immigrants. One of the largest groups in this mix are those immigrants from Mexico. Of particular concern is the adaptation of Mexican and other Latino immigrants who come to this country without documentation. Social workers have an ethical responsibility to serve these clients in a culturally competent and informed manner. They must keep updated on immigration policy and entitlement or eligibility issues that mitigate these immigrants' ability to survive. *[Article copies available for a fee from The Haworth Document Delivery Service: 1-800-HAWORTH. E-mail address: <docdelivery@haworthpress.com> Website: <http://www.HaworthPress. com> © 2004 by The Haworth Press, Inc. All rights reserved.]*

KEYWORDS. Mexican immigration, migration, immigration, undocumented immigrants

Maria Zuniga is Professor Emeritus, San Diego State University.

[Haworth co-indexing entry note]: "Mexican Immigrants: 'Would You Sacrifice Your Life for a Job?'" Zuniga, Maria. Co-published simultaneously in *Journal of Immigrant & Refugee Services* (The Haworth Social Work Practice Press, an imprint of The Haworth Press) Vol. 2, No. 1/2, 2004, pp. 119-138; and: *Immigrants and Social Work: Thinking Beyond the Borders of the United States* (ed: Diane Drachman, and Ana Paulino) The Haworth Social Work Practice Press, an imprint of The Haworth Press, Inc., 2004, pp. 119-138. Single or multiple copies of this article are available for a fee from The Haworth Document Delivery Service [1-800-HAWORTH, 9:00 a.m. - 5:00 p.m. (EST). E-mail address: docdelivery@haworthpress.com].

Latino immigrants who settle in the United States (U.S.) encounter experiences that are similar to most immigrants. These include the processes of how decisions are made to immigrate (Sluzki, 1979), the stressors endured during the immigration, the grief and loss related to leaving their relatives and familiar surroundings, and the stressors of learning how to cope in this new country, with its unique culture and English language (Drachman, 1992; Padilla, 1999). Themes that are particularly unique to Latino immigrants who enter the United States without documentation are the psychological and physical risks they endure in their immigration routes to seek jobs. For those who cross the U.S. Mexican border in the Southwest, Operation Gatekeeper, has impacted this already treacherous crossing (Annerino, 1999). The federal government has invested millions of dollars in sensor equipment, extended policing by the border patrol, and constructed new fences and light devices that insure detection. Consequently, those who immigrate without documents select out crossing areas that are now very dangerous but may result in successful journeys. One of these areas is the extensively polluted New River, near Calexico, California. This river has a steady stream of urban sewage, farm runoff and " . . . some of the most virulent diseases known to mankind" (Gross, 2000). In the San Diego/Imperial Valley region, immigrants have moved their crossings to the east, traversing major mountainous terrain at the risk of freezing in the winter. This area is also surrounded with extensive desert that has resulted in the deaths of hundreds of immigrants since the implementation of Operation Gatekeeper in 1994. Moreover, many immigrants now attempt to cross at sites located in desolate areas of Arizona. A photojournalist, John Annerino has highlighted these fateful journeys from the deserts of Mexico to the deserts of Arizona. He traversed "El Camino del Diablo," The Road of the Devil, which is the infamous historical route that resulted in the deaths of many Spanish colonizers, and today is the killing field for those immigrants from El Salvador, Nicaragua, Guatemala and Mexico (Annerino, 1999).

A unique overlay to these experiences is the reality that the Border Patrol's track record on abuses to immigrants is tarnished; on average there is at least one complaint lodged against agents on a daily basis (60 Minutes, 2001). As noted in the 60 Minutes journal program, this type of complaint record is unheard of in any other policing agency (60 Minutes, 2001). Such organizations as the American Friends Service Committee has undertaken interviews to identify border crossing abuse by the Border Patrol, documenting an array of abuses from verbal mistreatment to violent attacks, rapes, or even deaths of sojourners (Martinez, April 18, 2002).

Therefore, the experiences with immigration for Latino immigrants may include the unique trauma realities that correspond to undocumented status and the possibility of abuse from officials of the U.S. government. In addition, it is well known that "coyotes" or those who traffic in taking undocumented immigrants across, often desert them in the most life-threatening circumstances. Many other immigrants are attacked, robbed, or raped by Mexican border bandits. These experiences contribute to the kinds of trauma that can result in Post Traumatic Stress Syndrome. This syndrome should be one aspect of the assessment workers should undertake working with these immigrants (Perez-Foster, 2001; Zuniga, 2000). For other immigrants, witnessing the death of a family member due to the elements remains a helpless, guilt-ridden traumatic burden that burrows into their psyche. Annerino documents some of these horrible deaths of family members, including children (Annerino, 1999).

This chapter will examine some of the traditional themes related to the immigration experience for Latinos with documentation, with the major focus on the challenging experiences of those who are undocumented immigrants. Although the implications are relevant to undocumented immigrants from all Central and South American countries, the major emphasis for this paper is on the largest immigrating group, those from Mexico. The goal of the chapter is to inform social workers or human service workers of the special areas they must assess to insure they utilize this information and these insights in the design of their interventions. Whether an immigrant is documented or not, workers must be cognizant of the social policies that dictate which social or health services they can utilize without penalty and which, if utilized, may result in detection and deportation for those undocumented, or may inhibit other immigration proceedings for those who are documented.

DEMOGRAPHIC REALITIES

It is noteworthy that immigrants from Mexico are viewed by many people in the United States to rank near the bottom in terms of how Americans view immigrants from different parts of the world (Reimers, 1998). Given the September 11 terrorist attacks, it would be of interest to note if those immigrants from Middle Eastern cultures now rank lower. Some of the negative views held towards Mexican immigrants may be tied to the flow of Mexican immigrants who enter this country outside the legal process. Some of this negativity may evolve from historical derision of this group that has been enduring, stemming from the U.S. Mexican War of 1848 (Acuna, 1972). Other contributors to this negative sentiment may also be linked to the cultural differences that become highlighted when U.S. residents encounter the lifestyle of these new immigrants (Reimers, 1998).

In the 1990's almost a million immigrants entered the United States through legal means and at least 270,000 entered without documentation. At least 20 percent of legal immigrants and 67 percent of undocumented immigrants come from Mexico alone (Lindsay & Michaelidis, 2001). Presently, one in every ten Americans is foreign-born. However, in contrast to the major immigration epic of the 1930's where the majority of immigrants were from Europe, this present immigration epoch highlights patterns of immigration from Latino America, Asia, and other third world nations like Africa. Some of the anti-immigration sentiments of the last decade are based on the cultural differences that result from this diverse immigration (Reimers, 1998).

It is difficult to provide correct estimates of the numbers of immigrants who are in the United States without legal entry. There are three major ways that these persons become undocumented. The first class compose those who cross U.S. borders like those between the U.S. and Mexico or Canada, without detection by the Border Patrol. The second class are those who may have temporary visas to be in the U.S. as a student or tourist but continued to remain once their visa is expired. The third class are foreign nationals who may violate the conditions of their visas, for example, by taking a job when their visa had only been for the purpose of their tourism. About 40 percent of all undocumented immigrants are composed of those who overstay or violate their visas (Duigman & Gann, 1998). It is difficult to discern how many in this last group are composed of Mexican immigrants.

Latinos compose about two-thirds of the undocumented group. Those from Mexico compose more than 50 percent of this group with El Salvador making up 6.7 percent and Guatemala about 3.3 percent (Smith & Edmonston, 1997). The numerical count of all immigrants in the U.S. without documents is 5,000,000. For Mexico this count is 2,700,000, El Salvador 335,000, and Guatemala 165,000. In 1996 the states of residence for this undocumented population included California with 2,000,000; Texas with 700,000; New York with 540,000; Florida with 350,000; and Illinois with 290,000. The current estimates based on the early review of the 2000 Census placed the number of undocumented living in the U.S. even higher than the number noted above; between seven to eight million (Gonzalez, 2001).

Data from the Center for Immigration Studies, based on census figures, report that although Latino immigrants compose 12.8 percent of the work force, they are heavily concentrated in low-skill, low-paying jobs. Most of them have only a high school education or less (Kreisher, 2001). Yet this last census count and Labor Department data have provided some fascinating perspectives on the immigration issue, particularly the role of undocumented workers. These data indicate that undocumented workers have played a significant role in the growth of the New Economy. This New Economy of the 1990's had been linked mainly to high-tech job growth. However, this growth spawned a second tier of low-wage jobs in the service sector. These jobs were filled by undocumented workers as noted by a study by Northeastern University's Center for Labor Market Studies (Gonzalez, 2001). Unfortunately, many of these kinds of jobs could be eliminated in an economic downturn.

THE IMPACTS FROM THE 9-11-01 TERRORISM

The terrorist events of 9-11-01 have dramatically affected the economy of the United States, contributing to an economic downturn that had seemed to have already begun before 9-11-01. Although it is difficult to document the effect this has had on Latino immigrants, especially those here without documentation, it is obvious that the dramatic downturn of tourism has impacted them on a grand scale. In illustration, after 9-11-01, hotels and restaurants in San Diego, California, which cater heavily to tourism, were forced to lay off personnel due to tourist cancellations. The low level positions in these industries are filled by personnel who are largely Latino, many of whom are undocumented. This sad reality compelled the California Faculty Association at San Diego State University to request food donations and money to be given to the San Diego-Imperial Counties Labor Council Food Bank for those workers who had lost their jobs due to the terrorism. Since many of these were Mexicans who were undocumented, it was recognized that these immigrants had no union or other resources on which to rely.

Another impact of the terrorist event of 9-11-01 was on those Mexican nationals who worked in the twin towers in the many low-end jobs in the Towers' restaurants and cleaning services. During the initial days after the attack, Mexican television referred to these nationals, noting there was no way to ascertain an exact count of those employed at the

Towers or killed by the attack. Many of these immigrants were from Puebla, Mexico, highlighting the process of immigrants settling in sites where their relatives or friends have established networks. An agency called Casa Puebla, which is situated in New York City, was a resource for the numerous immigrants from Puebla. It now attempts to help relatives sort through information on the Twin Towers' dead or missing (Personal communication, Juarez, 2001).

One of the major sources of revenue for Mexico comes from the millions of dollars sent home by immigrants. Undoubtedly the economic downturn has effected both those individual families who no longer are in receipt of financial help from their relatives in the U.S. as well as the general economy of Mexico. A recent interview of the manager of a building supply business in Rosarito, Baja California, Mexico, indicated that his business has continued to be affected by 9/11. Since Baja California is home to many U.S. retirees, the normal home construction for these people that had occurred before 9/11 stopped abruptly after this event, affecting his business. Moreover, this has increased the unemployment of the construction workers in the surrounding towns, who survive on the building needs of American retirees. His business was also affected adversely by the U.S.- Iraqi War, when again, building requests by U.S. citizens who find it more economical to live in Mexico dropped dramatically (Pino H., 7-20-03).

The economic relationship between those immigrants who work in the U.S. and send money to their relatives in Mexico and the economic forces in the United States is both sensitive and tenuous (Engstrom, 2000). U.S. economic downturns typically mean greater unemployment for those, like these immigrants in lower end jobs which then affect their families in Mexico. These immigrants begin sending home less or no money at all. Many times, the immigrants in the U.S. are not able to maintain their own subsistence, often relying on private sources of aid like food banks from churches or non-government sources. Or others, who may still be working, may send home even more money, fearing that unemployment may be soon upon them.

Additionally, business in Mexico is also affected, especially in border towns that rely heavily on tourists for day shopping, such as those in Texas, Arizona, New Mexico and California. Moreover, since tourism is such a major income producer for Mexico, those U.S. tourists who became fearful of traveling, especially by air after 9-11 also resulted in a major negative impact on the tourist economy in Mexico (Gringo News, 2003.) These economic realities have added to the pressure on the president of Mexico, Vicente Fox, to advocate for a better immigration policy with President Bush, so as to relieve the economic stress that continues in Mexico. Mexico's recent election, in July, 2003, resulted in a dramatic loss of congressional seats of elected officials from Fox's Pan party, reflecting the disappointment of many Mexicans in President Fox's leadership and the continued economic downturns that Mexico faces.

GEOGRAPHIC TRENDS

The presence of Mexican immigrants at the Twin Towers Terrorism speaks to the recent trend of Mexican immigrants to locate in areas of the country outside of the normal Southwest region. For example, states like North and South Carolina, Virginia, and Tennessee have experienced dramatic increases in Mexican immigrants who are drawn to certain employment magnets, like the poultry packing houses in South Carolina. In illustration, during the last decade Arkansas experienced more than a 300 percent increase in Latino, and mainly Mexican immigrants; Alabama's increase was 208 percent; North Carolina's was 394 percent and Georgia's was 300 percent (*www.Census*, 2000). Historically, Mexican immigrants have flowed to those cities where migration networks have been established. Kin and friendship ties have typically been the most effective pathway for guiding new arrivals to those ethnic communities that have been established for many years (Engstrom, 2000). However, in the last decade there have been forays by some immigrant pioneers to newer settlement sites, and soon cousins or paesanos from their towns have been recruited by these countrymen to join them. This new migration had also been occurring in New York, resulting in the Twin Tower reality. These new migration patterns challenges social workers in those areas to learn how to intervene with these immigrants in a culturally competent manner.

THE EFFECTS OF ANTI-IMMIGRANT SENTIMENTS

In general, polls taken during the 1990's in different areas of the country have shown increased sentiment against immigration. In the 1994 California election where Proposition 187 was a success, a major motif that underpinned this proposition's passage was the belief that Latino immigrants, especially those not documented, were asserted to be a drain on the taxpayer (Reimers, 1998). This proposition was written to bar

undocumented residents from receiving welfare and educational benefits. It prohibited those without documentation from obtaining access to
the state's public educational systems, non-emergency medical care,
and cash benefits. Another provision of this proposition was that service
providers would be required to report persons suspected of being in the
U.S. without documents to the California Attorney General and the Immigration and Naturalization Service (INS). This public policy battle
was supported by Euro-Americans. Yet, this proposition was opposed
by most mainline religious and educational groups. The Catholic Church
in California stood against this proposition, yet many individuals who
were Catholic were for it (Reimers, 1998). This anti-immigrant sentiment was not just confined to California. Even African Americans began
to publicly state their opposition to immigration, especially in such areas as
Florida and New York (Reimers, 1998). Their argument was that Latino
immigrants were taking employment positions from poor African Americans. Although Proposition 187 was passed, it was immediately challenged
in the courts when Judge Mariana Pfaelzer ruled that it was unconstitu-
tional since it denied education to those here without documents, amongst
other reasons. Thus injunctions against it continue; it has never been implemented (Delaet, 2000).

The legislation, AB 540, presented to the California legislature is an
intriguing counter to proposition 187. In this legislation, those students,
who have resided in California without legal documents, would be allowed to enter California's public college/university systems, without
having to pay tuition at the price of out of state residents. California's
State University system's rate for out of state residents at the time of this
legislation in 2001 was $7,380 versus in-state tuition of $1,839; for the
University of California system which includes such schools as the University of California at Los Angeles or at Berkeley, the price was in excess of $10,000. These prices would prevent students from these poor
immigrant families from attending institutions of higher education. Liz
Guillen from Maldef, the Mexican American Legal Defense and Education Fund, worked to organize a pro-Latino camp to petition their legislators to vote for this bill, as evidenced by scores of emails sent to alert
Latinos/as in higher education (Chicle, 2001). The argument stated that
these students had made California their home. Since they came to the
United States with their parents, many have had little or no contact with
their birth country and had no intention of returning to Mexico. They
had satisfied California's academic requirements, and some had been
admitted to California's most prestigious universities. Like all U.S. citizens and legal residents, their parents had paid state sales and state and

federal income taxes. Thus, these immigrant students should be able to benefit from their parents' hard work and fiscal contributions to the state of California. This bill was passed in the California legislature in November, 2001. However, undocumented students are still not eligible for federal or state financial aid administered through the California Student Aid Commission (Cal Grants), (National Immigration Law Center, 1995). Although the act was passed, there continues to be a lack of clarity on how the University of California system will implement the bill.

This latter piece of legislation illustrates, the fluidity of the immigration dilemma, establishing access to higher education for those who are not documented just seven years after the passage of Proposition 187. Another illustration of this immigration fluidity is the more recent stance taken by unions, supporting immigration in spite of holding very rigid sentiments against immigrants less than 20 years ago (Reimers, 1998). With dwindling union membership, immigration holds hope of new recruitment sources.

HISTORICAL PERSPECTIVES

Mexico's economic realities have been the major push factor in sending immigrants to the United States. Historically, the lack of manpower during such episodes as World War II, have been some of the pull factors that eventually contributed to such immigration policies as the Bracero Program of the 1950s. Lack of manpower in the U.S. farming industry offered access to Mexican farm workers (Engstrom, 2000).

The lack of employment opportunities for the poor and for those Mexicans from small agricultural towns has continued the flow of Mexican immigration, both legal and undocumented to the U.S. The passage of IRCA, the Immigration Reform and Control Act of 1986, was argued to be the answer for reducing undocumented immigration from Mexico. It legalized those immigrants who had resided in the U.S. continuously prior to and after January 1, 1982. Individuals who were not felons, nor had three or more misdemeanors, were eligible to become citizens. It also offered employer sanctions, making it illegal for all employers to knowingly hire or recruit immigrants unauthorized to work in the United States. The arguments for support of this legislation was that this form of amnesty would result in the decline of undocumented workers who would consider the employer sanctions piece of the legislation, cause for difficulty in finding or keeping employment. IRCA also promoted an "anti-discrimination measure" that noted that employment discrimination based on national origin or citizenship status was illegal.

Although initial reports highlighted this legislation's positive deterrence of illegal immigration, later data noted that it did not in fact serve as a major deterrent against illegal immigration. Surveys conducted in different Mexican communities that were known as major sources of immigration to the United States concluded the legislation had not mitigated the intent of emigrants to migrate illegally. Since 1990 I.N.S. apprehensions climbed to 1, 169, 939 and continue to rise (DeLaet, 2000).

The San Diego Police Department has issued a policy that clarifies to policy officers the extent of their role in reporting people to the INS they encounter who are not here legally. In illustration, this department indicates to its officers they are not to report persons who are here without documents who they encounter in their policing duties, unless it is a person who has committed a felony.

IMPLICATIONS OF RECENT IMMIGRATION POLICIES ON IMMIGRANTS

It is critical that social policy courses in schools of social work incorporate content on immigration policies due to the dramatic implications of these policies. For example, these policies affect an immigrant client or family's eligibility for life-sustaining resources. This content inclusion will also enable students to recognize the kinds of legislative advocacy that immigrants need. Importantly, it will re-orient social work students to the history of this profession which initially served immigrant populations during its formative years. The field of social work is now in a similar epoch where the needs of immigrants challenge social workers to serve them in a culturally competent and informed manner. Although the focus of this chapter is on Latino immigrants, immigrant policies are relevant for any immigrant population.

Similarly, courses like Human Behavior and practice must teach students how serving immigrant clients demands comprehension of how immigration affects human beings and their family systems. These effects will challenge workers to recognize and address the special practice implications that I will detail later. In practice classes Social Work students should be asked to examine their feelings about their work with clients who may not be documented. It is critical that they honestly evaluate their political sentiments about this sensitive issue. They must not allow their personal sentiments to convolute their professional obligations to provide persons in need with the resources for which they are eligible (Zuniga, 2001). Moreover, if their political sentiments are not recognized and addressed, these attitudes will undermine their work with immigrants, adding to the distrust and alienation these sojourners already experience. In this following section I will offer some of the major recent policies that drive eligibility themes in human services. Students in a Human Behavior Courses taught by this author, identified various resources on legislation for Latino and other immigrants that are detailed in Appendix B, at the end of this paper. These resources will help to elucidate the specifics of the following policies that will be covered more generally (Betancourt et al., 2001).

THE ILLEGAL IMMIGRATION REFORM
AND IMMIGRANT RESPONSIBILITY ACT OF 1996

The difficulty in determining the extent Latino immigrants utilize welfare programs stems from the fact that many studies do not account for the ethnicity of immigrant welfare recipients. Some studies offer different estimates of the amount of welfare abuse, or if abuse actually exists (Engstrom, 2000). What was not difficult to determine during the 1990's was the substantive anti-immigration sentiment that had been building. During this time welfare reform was also a major policy priority for the Clinton administration. Thus, these two issues became intricately intertwined. Despite the lack of compelling evidence of widespread welfare exploitation by Latino immigrants, Congress passed the act noted above. It required that " . . . all family-based immigrants have an affidavit of support" from a sponsor before they enter the United States. The affidavit of support means that sponsors commit to supporting each petitioned immigrant at 125 percent of the poverty level. If individuals cannot meet this financial commitment, they are prevented from sponsoring family members as immigrants (Engstrom, 2000, p. 55). Public welfare agencies were held responsible for enforcing this affidavit of support requirement which became operational in 1997. The implications of this act, given the overrepresentation of Latinos in the ranks of the poor, are that many Latinos will be prevented from sponsoring relatives to come to the United States. This will have implications for continued separation of family members, especially the separation of children from their parents.

This act also addressed border control and enforcements. Resources were allocated for adding 6,600 new border patrol agents and staff. An important feature in this law was that battered spouses and children would be considered "qualified aliens" and thus eligible to receive public benefits, even if they are not documented. However, the abusing spouse must be a citizen or a lawful permanent resident. Thus families where domestic violence is occurring have rights to resources for which they would not normally be eligible. Some of the requirements include demonstrating they are currently residing in the U.S.; they resided at some time in the U.S. with the citizen or legal permanent resident spouse; the abuse of the spouse or spouse's child occurred some time during the marriage, but not necessarily while the partners were living together or in the U.S. Such documentation of battering such as police reports and restraining orders help with this verification (Roberts, 1995).

The Personal Responsibility and Work Opportunity Reconciliation Act of 1996, resulted in TANF or the Temporary Assistance for Needy Families which replaced AFDC or Aid to Families of Dependent Children. Although regulations of this act are too substantive to be detailed here, the key provision related to immigrant benefits will be identified. In 1996, most non-citizens lost eligibility for SSI or Social Security Disability benefits; this was reversed in 1997, restoring benefits to those receiving them on August 22, 1996, or for those who were or would become disabled. Non-citizens became ineligible for Food Stamps; however, refugees and veterans were exempt. New immigrants who arrived after August 22, 1996 would be barred from any federal means-tested benefits for five years. This means they would be ineligible for TANF, food stamps, SSI, and Medicaid. Again refugees and veterans would be exempt. However, the 1997 supplemental appropriations law, P.L. 104-18 permits states to purchase federal food stamps to serve immigrants who lose their federal food stamp benefits (Morse et al., 1998). Thus, each state made a decision on whether they would offer federal food stamp benefits to the immigrants residing in their state.

If a worker is employed in a welfare/TANF dissemination agency, or what are local welfare offices, the administration officials at their site are responsible for providing the Immigration and Naturalization Service with the names and data on immigrants as a method of verifying statistical information according to federal law. Consequently, from the forms that workers fill out, data are compiled and reported. On an individual basis, however, workers are not mandated to report cases to authorities if they discover a person does not have legal documentation.

However, for some agencies like the Regional Centers in California, which are private, non-profit agencies, funded by state funds to serve children deemed to be disabled from birth to age 18, the main eligibility criteria is residence. The eligibility workers do not ask about whether the person is documented. Applicants only have to show through rental receipts or utility bills or other types of verification that they have resided in the area in which they seek services. Or hospitals like Children's Hospital in San Diego, which is a private, non-profit facility, will offer emergency services to undocumented immigrants. If extended hospitalization is needed they work with the resources in Mexico to make necessary referrals since these patients are not eligible for any kind of medical coverage. In some areas like San Diego, there are organizations like the Binational Border Health Organization that have identified resources and contact people on both sides of the border that help facilitate health and social service referrals for immigrants.

IMPLICATIONS FOR PRACTICE: DEVELOPING RELATIONSHIP

Reporting Undocumented Immigrants

It is critical that social workers know they are under no mandate to inform the Border Patrol or the Immigration and Naturalization Service of a client or clients who are not documented. In fact, the Social Work Code of Ethics, indicates that social workers facilitate access to needed services for human beings in need, rather than function as deterrents to this access (Zuniga, 2001).

If and when social workers are ever mandated to report their clients due to their undocumented status, the ethical conflicts surrounding this kind of predicament must be addressed by the National Association of Social Workers. Unfortunately, this kind of predicament may not be too far in the future. For example, in the state of Arizona, there is pending legislation (HB2609), which if passed, would require Child Protective Services (C.P.S.) workers to report any undocumented immigrants to the U.S. Immigration and Naturalization Service and notify police of any criminal activity. According to the acting director of the Division of Children Youth and Families in that state, C.P.S.' social workers already notify police whenever there is a report of abuse as part of the worker's role in protecting the child. However, this director felt that asking the worker to report to the INS was wrong; he viewed it as crossing over into a completely different role that is outside of the worker's purview (Thomsen, 2001).

Social workers must be cognizant that only the Federal government and its appointees, such as Border Patrol and Immigration and Naturalization officers, have the authority and mandate to identify, report, or detain immigrants who are here without legal papers (Engstrom, 2001). Social workers in state, county, or private agencies are not authorized to undertake this kind of reporting. This theme is underscored since in this writer's experiences, workers are often uninformed about their role. Many are often unconscious of their disdain for immigrants who are not documented, and how their attitudes sometime feed into the misconception that these immigrants should be reported, and that social workers are obligated to report (Engstrom, 2001). The rationale is often offered, "they are breaking the law so they should be arrested." This theme will be elucidated further in the section below.

This issue of the need to report persons who are not documented is so sensitive, that workers intervening with immigrants must be conscious of the issues of distrust and fear many of the clients experience. If immigrants have had encounters with officials in their own countries of origin that have been exploitative or brutal, they will be fearful of people in authority. This would be especially relevant in the case of immigrants from countries like Guatamala, El Salvador or Nicaragua which have had civil strife/wars; or for those immigrants who have suffered abuse at the hands of the U.S. Border Patrol. For those immigrants from Latino countries where war has been their experience, the possibility of post traumatic stress syndrome may impact their interpersonal relations as well as their ability to adapt in this new country (Perez-Foster, 2001).

Consequently, workers must imbue their interactions with them in such a manner that the immigrant feels the worker has a "good heart," is respectful, and is someone to be trusted. Workers must indicate at the right moment that they will not be informing the INS or Border Patrol services if the clients are undocumented. For some agencies like the Regional Center (in California, they provide services to children who have major disabilities) the question is not even broached. Often, by referring them to pragmatic resources such as food or immigration information services, immigrants may begin to develop a sense of trust in the worker. Immigrants who have suffered trauma or have been abused will be extra-sensitive to the behaviors of workers and the ambience of the social service agency. If workers feel resentful about persons who are not documented, the immigrant will be ultra-sensitive to this attitude and is liable not to return. Importantly, the workers' counter-transference then has mitigated his or her ability and ethical responsibility to connect a human being to the services that are deemed his or her natural right as highlighted in the profession's Code of Ethics.

ASSESSING ELIGIBILITY

The humanism necessary to establish a working relationship with immigrants who are fearful will enable the worker to determine who are undocumented in a family system so that appropriate resources can be identified. Making this determination may be necessary to assure that prospects for legal immigration do not become jeopardized. The worker may want to preface their inquiry by highlighting the importance of keeping potential immigration eligibility open.

It is not unusual for children to be born in the United States while their parents might still be undocumented, although they have resided here for many years. These children are U.S. citizens by birth and eligible for social and health services. Yet their parents who are undocumented will be ineligible for Medicaid or other health services apart from such health measures as emergency medical care. Workers must identify such resources as Free Clinics or other private health care resources for such parents. In those cities where there are numerous immigrants, Church organizations often provide resources on immigration law, or food and clothing closets. Major churches like the Catholic, Lutheran, or Episcopal ministries enable immigrants to use their services without eligibility concerns. A sensitive issue, given the growing Protestant population both in Mexico and Latin America, is to insure to the applicant that referring them to a Catholic related service agency, for example, does not require one to be Catholic. Nor will the agency undertake any proselytizing effort.

Certainly, children who do not have documentation can be enrolled in school systems. Schools require that immunization records be current; immunization resources are provided by county services and are one of the services noted as necessary for public health needs, and thus an exception to the normal ineligibility for health care for those without documentation. Workers can utilize such private organizations like Boys Scouts or YMCA's to make referrals for recreational or other resources for teens or children without documentation.

ASSESSING FOR EXPLOITATION

Another area of concern is to assess for exploitation. Persons who live and work in this country without documents will often not report incidents to the police or authorities for fear of deportation. Workers need to evaluate if there are systems in their life, like their employment or housing, where they are being exploited. The use of Legal Aid or other avenues for advocating for their rights as human beings must be used by workers to mitigate exploitation. Some landlords have been known to charge excessive rent, but will not correct plumbing or even hazardous conditions since they know immigrants will not report them to authorities. The worker must realistically evaluate if advocacy efforts might even place them in greater jeopardy.

MENTAL HEALTH SERVICES

Immigrants who have suffered trauma must be helped to seek the counseling that will enable them to address trauma concerns as an avenue for insuring more effective adjustment. Thus, workers must differentiate the immigrant who is striving to adapt given the typical barriers that are encountered versus the immigrant who is overwhelmed by trauma issues who must also attempt to overcome typical immigration barriers that for them, may become insurmountable. Asking what country the immigrant is from informs the worker if the client is from a country with recent civil war history; thus, the worker must pursue questions that assess for trauma experiences.

For immigrants from Mexico who are not undocumented, workers must assess what their crossing experiences were like and what kind of trauma was experienced and at whose hands. To be the victim of trauma by a border bandit is difficult enough; to be traumatized by a Border Patrol Agent who one expects to be professional may color the trauma experience in a more painful hue.

Perez-Foster (2001) highlights several questions that the mental health worker should consider: "Does the trauma of war and disaster permanently impair the human psyche? Do people ever recover from psychological and physical torture? How do clinicians intervene so that people ultimately adjust to new host environments, and move on with productive lives?" (pp. 153-154). Professionals like Perez-Foster and others such as Espino (1991), Melville and Lykes (1992) and Mancilla (1987), provide insights on how Latino children, teens, and adults adapt as immigrants when trauma has been part of their experiences. Workers must become informed about these special themes by seeking out these readings.

Resource issues become a paramount problem for social workers since these clients will not be eligible for public mental health services. Again, private and typically church-sponsored agencies must be relied on for counseling services for these immigrants. In areas of the country like Portland, Oregon, which has a growing surge of Latino immigrants, community-based organizations have collaborated with churches in developing services for immigrants who cannot obtain resources in traditional agencies. The use of Promotoras or health educators who serve as supports, and facilitate groups that help families adapt to their new challenges contribute to resources that are linguistically and culturally appropriate. Since the Promotoras are immigrants themselves, some who have experienced trauma, clients may feel more comfortable in seeking their help. When professional services are not available, these kinds of alternative services may be the only remedy that can be utilized (Power in Partnership Conference, 2000).

CONCLUSION

The worker should not become overwhelmed with the range of knowledge they must develop if they are to serve Latino immigrants effectively. Appendix A provides various resources including sites where updates on legislation policy are available. Although resources are scarce, communities are attempting to find unique ways to address the issues that Latino immigrants face in the United States. As the recommended reading list in Appendix B notes, there is some beginning research on trauma and Latino immigrants. Workers must review this work to develop as much insight on this theme as possible to insure they do not overlook trauma history. In the south and mid west there are many community-based organizations that work to serve Latinos and in particular Latino immigrants. Contact with these agencies will help workers to discern what resources are available for undocumented clients. For those communities where Latino immigrants are newcomers, workers may need to work with governmental as well as private entities, as in the Portland, Oregon experience, to advocate on the part of these immigrants and to develop resources when resources are unavailable. Workers must assess their political sentiments to insure they do not maintain rejecting or hurtful attitudes towards Latino immigrants. They will also need to consult with service providers who are expert in serving Latino immigrants to upgrade their knowledge and skills. Learning about the immigration process and the particular adaptation stress immigrants experience will provide workers with a unique frame of reference. The Social Work profession committed itself to the needs of immigrants in past centuries. In this new century, we must re-commit ourselves to this new group of clients.

REFERENCES

Acuna, Rodolfo (1972). *Occupied America: The Chicano's struggle toward liberation.* San Francisco, Canfield Press.

Anneino, John. (1999). *Dead in their tracks: Crossing America's desert borderlands.* New York. Four Walls Eight Windows.

Betancourt, Sylvia, Maria Pilar Clark, Karina Corona, Zelalem Hagos, Michael Ostash (2001). Guide to Resources for working with Immigrants and their Families. *Social Work,* 619.

Chicle, *Chicle@linux08.UNM.EDU* Chicano literature discussion list, June 14, 2001.

Class on Human Behavior, San Diego State University, Fall, 2001.

Cowan, G., Martinez, L., & Mendiola, S. (1997). Predictors of attitudes toward illegal Latino immigrants. *Hispanic Journal of Behavioral Sciences,* Vol. 19, No. 4, November, 403-415.

DeLaet, Debra (2000). *U.S. Immigration Policy in an Age of Rights.* Praeger, Westport, Connecticut.

Drachman, D., & Halberstadt, A. (1992). A stage migration framework as applied to recent Soviet emigres. *Journal of Multicultural Social Work,* 2(1), 63-77.

Duignan, Peter, & Lewis H. Gann (Eds.) *The Debate in the United States over immigration.* Stanford, CA: Hoover Institution Press, 1998.

Engstrom, David. (2000). Hispanic Immigration at the New Millennium. Pastora San Juan Cafferty and David Engstrom, (Eds.) *Hispanics in the United States: An Agenda for the Twenty-First Century.* Transaction. New Brunswick, pp. 31-68.

Engstrom, David. (2001). Personal communication, 11-28-01.

Espino, Conchita M. (1991). Trauma and Adaptation: The case of Central American children. In Frederick Ahearn and Jean Athey (Eds.) *Refugee Children: Theory, Research, and Services.* (p. 67-85) Baltimore: Johns Hopkins University Press.

Gonzalez, Daniel. Illegal workers fueled New Economy, study says. *The Arizona Republic,* February 19, 2001.

Gross, Gregory Alan. (2000). Immigrants navigate the contaminated New River every day in a desperate attempt to enter the U.S. *San Diego Union-Tribune.* March 12. A-1.

Immigration Legal Resource Center. Naturalization: A guide for legal practitioners and other community advocates. San Francisco, CA. Immigration Legal Resource Center.

Kreisher, Otto (2001). Poor immigrants growing presence in state, union. *San Diego Union Tribune.* Friday, January 5, Page A9.

Lindsay, James, & Michaelidis, M. (2001). A timid silence on American's immigration challenge. *San Diego Union Tribune,* January, 5, B7.

Los Angeles Times, November 20, 1994. P. 25, Roberts, Maurice, Editor-in-Chief. (1995). Interpreter Releases (ISSN 0020-9686). Report and analysis of immigration and nationality law. Vol. 72, No. 14, April 10, Federal Publications Inc., Washington, D.C.

Mancilla, Y.E. (1987). Exposure to war-related violence and psychosocial competence of adolescent males from El Salvador, Unpublished manuscript.

Martinez-Perez, Isidro. Personal Communication, 11-12-01.

Martinez, Roberto. (April 18, 2002). Personal communication with the former director of the American Friends Committee in San Diego, CA.

Melville, M.B., & Lykes, M.B. (1992). Guatemalan Indian children and the sociocultural effects of government-sponsored terrorism. *Social Science and Medicine*, 34, 533-548.

Morse, Ann, Jeremy Meadows, Kirsten Rasmussen, Sheri Steisel (1998). America's Newcomers: Mending the Safety Net for Immigrants. National Conference of State Legislatures, Washington, D.C.

National Immigration Law Center (February, 1995). Immigrants' Rights Brief Answers to Common Question. Los Angeles, California.

Padilla, Yolanda. (1999). Immigrant Policy: Issues for social work practice. In P.L. Ewalt, E.M. Freeman, A.E. Fortune, D.L. Poole, & S. Witkin (Eds). *Multicultural Issues in Social Work: Practice and Research*. (pp. 589-604). Washington, DC: NASW.

Perez-Foster, Rose Marie (2001j). When immigration is trauma: Guidelines for the individual and family clinician. *American Journal of Orthopsychiatry*, 71(1). April. 153-170.

Pino, Horatio. Personal communication, July 20, 2003. Power in Partnership Conference (2000) Coordinated by Lorena Connelly, Marie Dahlstrom, Catherine Fixe, Colleen Keyes & Lucrecia Suarez. University of Portland, Portland Oregon.

Reimers, David. (1998). *Unwelcome Strangers: American Identity and the Turn Against Immigration*. Columbia University Press, New York.

60 Minutes, The U.S. Border Patrol. Sunday, November 28, 2001.

Sluzki, Carlos. (1979). Migration and family conflict. *Family Process*. 18. 379-390.

Smith, James P., & Barry Edmonston (Eds). (1997). *The New Americans: Economic, Demographic, and Fiscal Effects of Immigration*, Washington, D.C.: National Academy Press.

Thomsen, Scott (2001). *Bill would require CPS social workers to turn in illegal immigrants*. The Associated Press, February 20.

www.census, 2000

Zuniga, Maria (2001). Latino Immigrants in Rowena Fong and Sharon Furuto (Eds). *Cultural Competent Practice: Skills, Interventions, and Evaluations*. (p. 47-60). Boston, MA: Allyn & Bacon.

APPENDIX A
Information Resources

1. What are my true sentiments about undocumented immigrants? See this article to discuss the various ways these attitudes develop: Cowan, G., Martinez, L. & Mendiola, S. (1997). Predictors of Attitudes Toward Illegal Latino Immigrants. *Hispanic Journal of Behavioral Sciences*, Vol. 19 No. 4, November, 403-415.
2. Who could give me information on the rights of immigrants? In California the Coalition or Humane Immigrants Rights of Los Angeles offers relevant data. (888) 624 4752.
3. If I was trying to advocate for a client who is an immigrant worker being exploited by his employer, who might I call? Office of Special Counsel (OSC) (800) 255:7688.
4. I am clueless about the naturalization process. How can I learn more without having to read legal jargonese? Written for the non-attorney, this guide provides detailed information on naturalization: Naturalization: A Guide for Legal Practitioners and Other Community Advocates. Immigration Legal Resource Center, 1663 Mission St., Suite 602, San Francisco, CA. 94103. (415) 225-9499 (415) 225:9792 (fax).
5. Also, a website at <*www.ilw.com/wernick/*> offers resources on immigration and citizenship.
6. <*http://<www.nclr.org*> The National Council of La Raza (NCLR) is a private, nonprofit, nonpartisan tax-exempt organization established in 1968. It has a policy department that has the most current updates on immigration legislation.*
7. <*http://<ncpa.org*> The National Center of Policy Analysis (NCPA) is a nonprofit, nonpartisan public policy research organization.*
8. <*http://<www.cis.org*> This is the home page for the Department of Immigration and Naturalization Services.*

APPENDIX B
Suggested Readings
(* THESE ARE RESOURCES NOTED BY BETANCOURT ET AL.)

- Annerino, John. (1999). Dead in their tracks: Crossing America's desert borderlands. New York: Four Walls Eight Windows.
- Arbruster, R., Geron, K., Bonacich, E. (1995).The Assault on California's Latino Immigrants: The Politics of Proposition 187. Cambridge, MA. Blackwell Publishers.*
- Chavez, L.R. (1992). Shadowed Lives: Undocumented Immigrants in American Society. New York, NY: Harcourt Brace Jovanovich College Publishers.*
- Fix, M., & W. Zimmerman. (1999). All Under One Roof: Mixed-Status Families in an Era of Reform. Washington, DC: The Urban Institute.*

An East-West Approach
to Serving Chinese Immigrants
in a Mental Health Setting

Irene Chung
Florence Samperi

SUMMARY. This article discusses the unique design of a community day treatment program that addresses the issues of loss and acculturation for a Chinese American immigrant population who suffers from chronic mental illness. The program utilizes an integrated, multi-cultural milieu of staff and clients to create a microcosm of the diversity of American society, and reflects the agency's belief in the affirmation of the clients' cultural heritage as a more effective way of supporting clients in their recovery process. Case vignettes are used to illustrate the importance of helping immigrant clients who are marginalized in society to feel accepted, empowered and hopeful in their lives in a new country. *[Article copies available for a fee from The Haworth Document Delivery Service: 1-800-HAWORTH. E-mail address: <docdelivery@haworthpress.com> Website: <http://www.HaworthPress.com> © 2004 by The Haworth Press, Inc. All rights reserved.]*

Irene Chung, PhD, CSW, is Assistant Professor, Hunter College School of Social Work, City University of New York.

Florence Samperi, CSW, is Co-Administrative Director and Director of Training, Community Consultation Center, Henry Street Settlement.

[Haworth co-indexing entry note]: "An East-West Approach to Serving Chinese Immigrants in a Mental Health Setting." Chung, Irene, and Florence Samperi. Co-published simultaneously in *Journal of Immigrant & Refugee Services* (The Haworth Social Work Practice Press, an imprint of The Haworth Press) Vol. 2, No. 1/2, 2004, pp. 139-159; and: *Immigrants and Social Work: Thinking Beyond the Borders of the United States* (ed: Diane Drachman, and Ana Paulino) The Haworth Social Work Practice Press, an imprint of The Haworth Press, Inc., 2004, pp. 139-159. Single or multiple copies of this article are available for a fee from The Haworth Document Delivery Service [1-800-HAWORTH, 9:00 a.m. - 5:00 p.m. (EST). E-mail address: docdelivery@haworthpress.com].

http://www.haworthpress.com/web/JIRS
Digital Object Identifier: 10.1300/J191v02n01_09

KEYWORDS. Chinese immigrants, immigration, migration, mental health, community mental health

INTRODUCTION

Since the passage of the Immigration Act in 1965, which drastically altered the restrictive quota system based on race, Asian Americans have become one of the fastest growing immigrant groups in the United States (U.S.) (Uba, 1994). According to the U.S. Census Bureau, the Asian American population increased by 107.8 percent (from 3.5 million to over 7 million) between 1980 and 1990. Between 1990 and 1998, Asians and Pacific Islanders had the highest rate of population growth than any other race or ethnic group. In 1997, sixty percent of Asian Americans were immigrants.

With the influx of Asian immigrants, there has been an increased demand for culturally competent mental health services for this population. As an ethnic minority group, the stressors of readjustment and racism in a Western society have greatly increased Asian American immigrants' vulnerability to mental health risk. However, Asian Americans have always been noted for their underutilization of mental health services due to the cultural stigma associated with mental illness and the lack of culturally sensitive services (McNeil & Kennedy, 1997; Uba, 1994). In New York City, a major hub for Asian immigrants, mental health clinics serving this population are constantly grappling with the issues of non-compliance of treatment and recidivism among the chronically mental ill clients (personal interviews with administrators and staff of several major mental health clinics in the Asian community in NYC, August 2002).

This article will discuss the needs of a segment of the Asian immigrant population who suffers from mental illness from a psychological, social and cultural perspective and the unique design of a community program that addresses those needs. The authors posit that the loss of one's identity that is associated with migration and impacted by mental illness is the main underlying problem affecting this population. The article will discuss how a community program seeks to address this problem using a multi-cultural milieu that fosters a sense of hope and integration for the immigrant clients.

COMMUNITY CONSULTATION CENTER

Community Consultation Center (CCC) is a mental health clinic under the auspices of Henry Street Settlement, which has a long history of serving new immigrants from all over the world. Located on the Lower East Side of New York City, CCC provides mental health services to a diverse ethnic clientele that includes African Americans, Hispanics and Chinese Americans. Over the past six years, the Chinese clientele at CCC has grown rapidly. Presently, over fifty percent of the clientele at the Day Treatment Program of CCC is of Chinese descent.

Profile of Clients

The clientele at CCC could be considered as having the most adjustment difficulties and the least resources among the immigrant population. The majority of them are first-generation young and middle-aged immigrants who are monolingual with limited educational and employment history in this country. They are recent immigrants who came to the U.S. during the past ten years. Being single with limited job skills, most live with their families in tight quarters and rely on them for support and assistance. There is also a growing undocumented clientele who resides in boarding houses or receives temporary housing from relatives and friends. All of them carry serious psychiatric diagnoses such as schizophrenia, major depression with psychotic features and bipolar disorder, and require strict adherence to psychotropic medication to manage their symptoms.

Stories of Migration and Resettlement

Like most immigrants, the majority of the Chinese clients immigrated to the United States primarily for social, economic and political reasons (Drachman 1992). Most come from rural areas or fishing villages in China to seek a better quality of life. Some of them came with their families when they were adolescents; others came to join their families as young adults. They left behind grandparents and other members of their extended families, who have often developed close ties with them as their surrogate parents when they were infants and young children.

To the clients and their families who experienced the political chaos and economic hard times of the Cultural Revolution in the late sixties, leaving their home country has bittersweet significance. In interviews with the clinic staff, clients discussed their mixed feelings around their migration to the U.S. On one hand, they feel fortunate to be able to start a new promising life and forget the painful past. Having the resources and/or opportunity to leave for the United States is generally considered to be a prestigious feat and an issue that evokes envy in the homeland.

Thus, despite having to pay the emotional price of leaving behind one's family ties and heritage, one never feels that one could turn down the opportunity to emigrate. On the other hand, there is the grim reality upon arrival in the U.S. that one has to pay off the huge loan of fees and travel expenses, and there is great pressure and expectation to establish oneself successfully in the new country.

Among these Chinese clients, there is often an implicit pact that one cannot return to China until one has gained sufficient status and wealth in this country. Hardships and emotional pains are to be endured silently, as befitting with Asian cultural values (Ross-Sheriff, 1992; Uba, 1994). Akhtar (1995) compares these immigrants who cannot easily and frequently visit their home country to those in exile, and he describes their pain as being "barred from emotional refueling" (p. 1054). For many Chinese clients and their families, returning to China for retirement and reunion with their families is their ultimate goal. They view their emigration to the U.S. as a transitory journey to build their assets and provide for their families in China. Hsu (1971) indicates that in the Chinese culture, family ties are roots and bonds that last throughout the immigrant's lifetime.

Given the aforementioned perspectives, the post migration experience of the clients at CCC is filled with stressors in coping with losses, failures, disappointments, and cultural shock (Akhtar, 1995; Ross-Sheriff, 1992, Uba, 1994). Their stories since their arrival in the U.S. are similar. Like other immigrants from a non-Western culture, their distinctly different language, physical features and life styles often create more prejudices and discrimination against them and made their assimilation into American society extremely difficult.

Initially these clients struggled with enrolling in schools or maintaining menial jobs in restaurants and garment factories. However, the onset or exacerbation of their mental illness changed the course of their struggles. Since then, the life of resettlement has become a cycle of futile employment and psychiatric hospitalizations. These clients could be considered as a "marginalized" group that has not been able to assimilate into American society and at the same time is alienated from their own ethnic support system because of their mental illness (Berry, 1984; Ross Sheriff, 1992).

Coping with Mental Illness and Pursuing the Immigrant's Dream

For most of the Chinese clients, work is a premium value and priority. Apart from the very practical issue of being financially sufficient for those who have no family support, employment, or employability, represents the hope that one could still fulfill the immigrant's dream in this land of opportunities. It is also their only hope to regain acceptance and approval from their families who often have very little understanding of the origin and nature of their mental illness.

Sue and Morishima (1982) cited studies that found Asian Americans commonly perceive emotional disturbance as symptoms that can be alleviated by the exercise of will power and avoidance of morbid thoughts. While the clients' feelings of disappointment and frustration toward their mental illness are often masked by their psychiatric symptoms and heavy medications, their families' reactions are often angry and negative. Given the stigma of mental illness in the Chinese culture (Uba, 1994), the clients' mental disability is a shameful occurrence that their families cannot bear to reveal to relatives at home. Also, clients have often revealed that their mental illness was perceived by their family as a condemnation of their leaving their home country as well as a bad omen of their hope to return. Thus, on many levels it is tremendously important for clients to demonstrate that they can secure and maintain employment.

Antithetical to this symbolic accomplishment of finding employment is the stark reality of the need for clients to take the time for recuperation and comply with treatment. Unfortunately, the lack of culturally sensitive personnel and treatment modalities has created a great deal of distrust and underutilization of the Western mental health system among the Chinese clientele (Owan, 1981; Wong, 1981; Uba, 1994). Oftentimes, Chinese clients complain of adverse side effects of Western psychotropic medication and are suspicious of its effectiveness. Conditions such as fatigue, drowsiness and rigidity of body movements as induced by the medication are often regarded as more dysfunctional than auditory delusions or paranoid ideations. Families often indicate that they can more readily tolerate clients' irrational beliefs and behavior than their inability to be productive in their endeavors. Subsequently, many clients, pressured by their families, are erratic in their adherence to their prescribed medication regimen. Yet in their desperation to improve their functioning, many of the clients experiment with herbal medicines, acupuncture treatment, superstitious practices, and even resort to the old folklore practice of entering into pre-arranged marriages with women and men in their homeland in the hope of "uplifting" and "changing over" their spirits. Often times, acupuncture treatment and herbal medicine may stabilize the clients' symptoms in varying degrees, but their effectiveness is also undermined by the clients' unwillingness to commit to a treatment regimen. As soon as their levels of functioning improve, clients will sabotage their recovery by returning to work prematurely.

The Philosophy and Service Design of Community Consultation Center: Hope, Growth and Integration

As a mental health clinic staffed primarily by professional social workers, Community Consultation Center upholds the social work values of respecting individual differences, as well as recognizing and maximizing the inner strengths of clients (Saleebey, 1996). As a community agency with a mission of serving newly arrived immigrants, Community Consultation Center believes that the affirmation of clients' ethnic identity and heritage is an important value that goes hand in hand with provisions of assistance in their acclimation to American society. For new immigrants who are afflicted by mental illness, CCC recognizes that the treatment process needs to address the feelings of hopelessness and their impoverished self-image around their migration that are accentuated by the chronic and stigmatized nature of their illness.

The following section will discuss how the program design of CCC's Continuing Day Treatment Program reflects a philosophical structure that fosters hope, growth and integration for an immigrant clientele that has encountered multiple obstacles in their resettlement efforts in this new country.

Affirmation of cultural identity and heritage. CCC's Continuing Day Treatment Program provides a therapeutic milieu where clients are respected for their different backgrounds and life experiences. It supports a treatment context that enables clients to take pride in their own cultural heritage and at the same time, develop openness to values of a new culture that can truly complement those of their countries of origin. Relationships among staff as well as between staff and clients are one of mutual respect and curiosity for each other's differences. Customs reflecting the cultures of the various ethnic clientele in the clinic are celebrated with clients' input and assistance.

According to Saleebey (1996), these are "cultural approaches to healing" for clients, which serve as "a source for the revival and renewal of energies and possibilities" (p. 299). For the Chinese clients, Mid-Autumn Festival and Chinese New Year are major holidays symbolizing harmony and prosperity within families. Having the opportunity to plan for the holidays and share folklores and customs about the holidays with other client groups have been empowering and therapeutic experiences for the Chinese clients. As Greene, Jensen, and Jones (1996) aptly point out, an essential component of the empowerment process is helping the client to become more connected to his or her ethnic identity.

Microcosm of the diversity of American society. Unlike other day treatment programs where the clientele is fairly homogenous, CCC's Program is a multi-ethnic community where participants can interact with a diverse ethnic clientele and learn about the complexities of American culture. Chinese clients who are recently admitted into the Program are encouraged to explore American culture through participation in activities and classes. This acculturation experience is unique in the sense that clients are not co-opted into the dominant culture. Greene, Jensen, and Jones (1996) underscore the detrimental effects on the self-esteem of members of minority groups when their ethnic attributes are being devalued by those in the majority.

Since all cultures are given equal credence in the Program, acculturation is more a reciprocal process and a transitional experience with a mix of the familiar and the new for clients. The variety of food that is served and consumed in the Program is a good case in point. At breakfast, it is not uncommon for Chinese clients to enjoy a hearty portion of scrambled eggs, oatmeal and toast, while other ethnic clients partake in Chinese buns and dim sum. Thanksgiving menu usually consists of egg rolls, Chinese dumplings, pernil with collard greens, rice and beans, along with the traditional turkey and all the trimmings. Also, in language classes, Chinese clients are paired with non-Chinese clients to tutor each other in Chinese and English. In theatre productions, Chinese clients will often sing in English, while non-Chinese clients will perform Chinese folk songs.

In all these program activities, clients are in the dual role of receiving and giving. There is a tremendous sense of pride and pleasure in being able to teach, learn, create, and share. The enhancement of self-esteem and self-image is immeasurable. For the Chinese clients, there is the additional psychological gain of feeling accepted in American society for the first time. Their positive experience in the Program validates their cultural heritage and reinforces the idea that they can maintain their roots and develop a bicultural identity. Most important of all, it rekindles their hope that someday they can become functional members of American society.

"Depathologizing" mental illness and reframing the treatment process. Since their enrollment in CCC's Day Treatment Program, the majority of the Chinese clients have been able to break the debilitating cycle of decompensation and recidivism, and make good progress in

stabilizing and managing their mental illness. (In the past five years, only two percent of the clients at CCC were rehospitalized, despite the fact that the majority of them had a history of multiple hospitalizations prior to their enrolment at CCC.) Such success is attributable to the approach of the Program and its staff in viewing the client as a "whole" person with unique qualities and a history that evolves around meaningful relationships with peers and family members. Mental illness is perceived and presented to clients as an "aberration" of life that is no different from any physical disability or chronic medical condition. The concept of recovery is recognized as having different meanings for clients and their families (Jacobson, 2001).

As mentioned earlier, work and productivity are synonymous to recovery among the Chinese clients and their families. Thus, the recommended treatment regimen entails a great deal beyond medication compliance. Chinese clients are specifically presented with the options of participating in vocational rehabilitation and skill-training activities. In return, staff time is committed to helping clients secure government entitlements, subsidized housing and medical care, as well as free medication for those who are not eligible for any government assistance. For the Chinese clients, normalizing the concept of mental illness, emphasizing the need for vocational rehabilitation, and the offering of concrete services are extremely important approaches in motivating them to comply with treatment. The promise of recovery and the alleviation of pressure to seek financial resources make the commitment to receive treatment a worthwhile investment. It is interesting to note that many clients and their families like to refer to the Program as a "school" and their daily participation in the Program as "attending classes."

Eliciting Family Involvement and Support

"The (Asian American) client should be understood in the context of his family" (Kim, 1981). CCC recognizes the central function of the family in Asian culture, and the crucial role that the values of affiliation and loyalty play in shaping one's identity and life goals (Lee, 1996). Very often, sanction from a Chinese client's family for their son or daughter to enroll in a Western treatment program is instrumental in that client's compliance with treatment and subsequent recovery. Hsu (1970) and Roland (1987) explain how the concept of self in Asian culture is a collective self in the context of relationships with others, and fulfilling one's emotional needs takes the form of conformity to group and familial wishes. This concept is very different from the Western concept of self, which emphasizes rugged individualism, independence and freedom over affective bonds.

The work of engaging the client's family begins at the intake process. Generally, parents, siblings or relatives who are caregivers of the client are invited to attend a family meeting with the Program Administrator and a bicultural staff team. The family session is strategically planned to give credence to the closeness of the family and the hardships it has endured migrating to a Western country. Stories about the family's emigration are elicited. Staff in turn speaks openly about their own family emigration experiences in regard to losses, separations and sacrifices.

The deliberate use of "self-disclosure" among the staff is effective in transcending potential power differentials between professionals from the dominant culture and clients from a minority immigrant culture. It forges a common ground for staff and clients, and underscores the often forgotten fact that clients and their families possess a great deal of inner strength and resources (Saleebey, 1996). The acknowledgement and acceptance of the families' pain and strength is therapeutic and empowering. Very often, silent tears as stories are being told and firm handshakes at the end are gestures that trusting bonds have been formed between the families and the staff. For families who have been closely involved with caring for clients, it is important that they feel comfortable entrusting the care of their loved ones into a Western program facility, and not view it as another potential loss in their lives.

Collaboration of multi-ethnic staff. CCC's staff team consists of Chinese staff as well as staff of African, Hispanic, Irish, Jewish, German, Sicilian and Syrian descent. The diverse ethnicity of the staff serves many therapeutic functions in the treatment milieu. They represent the old and the new worlds of the Chinese clients. Their presence and their roles in activities and sessions create different dynamics that are complementary toward helping clients develop the confidence in achieving a bicultural identity.

When Chinese patients in the hospital are referred to CCC as part of their discharge plans, the Coordinator of the Asian Bicultural Services makes a policy of visiting the Chinese clients in the hospital. This outreach strategy by a bilingual and bicultural Asian staff has been effective in ensuring that clients feel connected to the Program and follow through with their commitment to attend the Program after their discharge from the hospital.

At the intake session with the Chinese clients and their families, the presence of an Asian and non-Asian staff team represents an integration of Eastern and Western cultures in American society, which sets a positive tone for the meeting. The Administrator of the Program, who is non-Asian, plays the role of a traditional Chinese host and starts the meeting by offering tea to the client and the family. As the Asian staff initiates the introduction, the non-Asian staff offers apology for not speaking the Chinese language. These culturally sensitive gestures create a feeling of equanimity and genuine warmth between the staff and the family, and pave the way for the intimate sharing of migration stories mentioned in the preceding section. They also reinforce the perspective that the client's identity is, first and foremost, member of an immigrant family.

During the intake session (and subsequent family sessions), the non-Asian staff takes on the task of addressing the feelings of guilt and shame associated with having mental illness in the family. As representatives of the Western culture, their words of universalizing mental illness seem to make a better impact on the Chinese clients and their families. Their compliments on the positive attributes of the client also interject a more hopeful prognosis on his/her recovery. The Asian staff usually represents members of an extended family who understands the nuances of the Chinese family dynamics, and could be marshaled to offer support in the forms of clarification and mediation with the non-Asian staff. The intake session as co-hosted by Asian and non-Asian staff is symbolic of the transferencial image the Program wants to project to the Chinese clients and their families, i.e., a therapeutic "holding environment" (Winnicott, 1965, p. 47) that respects their cultural heritage and help them transition into American society based on individual choices and not co-option.

As Chinese clients begin their attendance in a new setting, their feelings of trepidation and ambivalence are alleviated by a sense of familiarity provided by the presence of the Asian staff and their support and orientation. As clients settle down in the Program, they feel more confident communicating in English with the non-Asian staff, and feel more accepted and empowered when staff shows genuine interest in learning their language and culture.

Individualized Seamless Service Plans

There are various service components in CCC's Day Treatment Program that clients can utilize as their needs and capabilities change in their course of treatment. These service components range from medication monitoring, individual and family counseling, advocacy and concrete services, pre-vocational and ESL (English as a Second Language) classes, VESID (Vocational and Educational Services for Individuals with Disability) training and job placement. CCC believes that it is vital that each client develops an individualized treatment plan and time frame that takes into consideration the client's ego functions, resources, family responsibilities and expectations (Jacobson, 2001). These services are organized around integrating a client's past, current and future life roles.

For the Chinese clients, individual and family counseling are important services that help to resolve past conflicts regarding family loyalty and individual differentiation. The foci of the sessions usually revolve around reframing the nature of the conflicts and reducing their toxicity (Greene, Jensen, & Jones, 1996), as well as setting short-term goals that alleviate individual stress and preserving the integrity of the family system. Coupled with concrete services that usually bring in resources and reinforces stability in the family, the Chinese client becomes more hopeful regarding his/her recovery and is more motivated to comply with his/her medication regimen, which in turn, enables him/her to enroll in classes and eventually vocational training. However, depending on the history and nature of the psychiatric illness as well as family dynamics, it is common that clients may encounter setbacks at different stages of their treatment. At such occurrence, client's assigned social worker will meet with client and his/her family to amend the treatment plan. The individualized seamless service plans offer a safety net for clients to move back and forth without experiencing a sense of failure.

CASE VIGNETTES

The following case vignettes are illustrations of CCC's Chinese immigrant clientele and the Program's treatment approaches. While the recovery process varied for each individual client, their stories of stabilization of symptoms and family relationships denote the common themes of hope and growth.

Wang

Wang entered this country illegally at aged thirty-three, incurring a smuggling fee of $20,000, which he tried to pay off by working long hours as a chef in a Chinese restaurant. Wang came from the fishing villages of Fu Jian, where unemployment abounds and many men have left for the United States in search of a better livelihood. Wang left behind his wife and three young children, whom he had no hope of reuniting with in the near future due to his illegal status. Wang had a cousin in New York City whom he called on infrequently. Wang spoke very little English and lived in a rented room in the Chinese community. A couple of years after arrival in this country, Wang began showing symptoms of mental decompensations. He was arrested several times for shoplifting and threatening behavior in department stores, and was subsequently hospitalized in a psychiatric unit of a City Hospital with a diagnosis of Psychosis NOS. For several years, Wang went through multiple hospitalizations, and eventually spent six months in a State Hospital before being referred to CCC for aftercare. Wang's psychiatric history revealed a pattern of acute hospitalizations, followed by erratic aftercare services that were interrupted by frantic attempts to seek employment.

At the intake session with Wang, the staff spent a great deal of time exploring Wang's stories of migration, his feelings around separation from his family and his financial obligations. Wang felt supported by the staff's sensitivity and concern, and was neither defensive nor resistant when the issue of his treatment plan came up. Wang agreed to attend CCC's Day Treatment five days a week for one month, during which time he would be monitored for his medication, take ESL classes, and meet with his counselor to discuss job options and any concrete services he might need. This one-month attendance at CCC was presented to Wang as prevocational training and consistent with his goal of returning to work. Since the plan was short-term and task-oriented, Wang abided by the agreement faithfully. The staff also extended themselves to maximize the therapeutic value of his brief, one-month attendance. Carfare, lunch money, and medications were procured from the State Hospital that discharged Wang to spare him from incurring any expenses. Phone calls were made to Wang in the morning if he was late in arriving at the Program. Efforts were made to introduce Wang to other Chinese clients who were in similar predicaments, especially those who came from the same province in China. Soon after, Wang became an active participant in the ESL class and the Asian Bicultural Group Discussion. At the end of one month, Wang was pleased with the completion of his attendance, his accomplishments in the various groups and activities, and his improved mental status. For the first time since his arrival in the U.S., Wang felt validated for his decision to emigrate and was hopeful that his family would someday benefit from his sacrifices. From a treatment perspective, the most valuable gains were Wang's acceptance of and insights into his mental illness, as well as the positive transference he has developed for the Program as a trusting transitional family that he could turn to for ongoing support. Wang resumed working after the first month. He took a job that was less demanding and he made a commitment to attend the Program weekly on his day off from his restaurant job. He took responsibilities to comply with his medication regimen, and understood the warning signs of "hearing voices." Despite his limited English, Wang approached the non-Asian administrators regularly to express his appreciation and to reassure them that he is doing well. On Chinese New Year, Wang took time off from work and came into the Program to help prepare an authentic Chinese meal. He demonstrated his culinary skills and made delicious fresh dumplings to serve all the clients and their families. Several months later, Wang contacted the staff and disclosed that he was under great distress because his wife had been arrested and detained by immigration officials for attempting to enter the U. S. illegally. The staff made phone calls on his behalf to the Immigration Office and Legal Aid Society. During this crisis, Wang managed his stress with the support from staff and clients at CCC, and did not suffer a relapse. Wang's wife was eventually released and both husband and wife were able to obtain legal aid to apply for legal immigrant status. Recently, Wang and his wife moved to another borough and he transferred to an outpatient clinic in his neighborhood. He also received his "green card," and is in the process of applying for visas for his children. Wang has made tremendous progress in his recovery and rebuilding his life as an immigrant in this country.

San

San came to the U.S. from Canton province with her father, stepmother, older sister and younger stepbrother at the age of fifteen. San spoke some English, but not fluently enough to keep up with the demands of high school. A year after her arrival, San was hospitalized for psychotic behavior and suicidal ideations. She was given a diagnosis of schizophrenia, and was subsequently hospitalized several times before she was referred to CCC for aftercare services. San's father and older sister came to the intake session with San. During the course of discussion about the family's life in China and its decision to emigrate, San's father revealed for the first time to his daughters that their biological mother was a victim of political persecution during the Cultural Revolution who committed suicide shortly after San's birth. To San's father, it was a big relief for him to be able to unburden the family secret. It also appeared that the gesture was symbolic of his willingness to entrust his daughter to the care of a staff that understood his past as well as his hopes for a new beginning for her. However, San's prognosis at the time was poor, given her history of multiple hospitalizations in a span of two years, and her depressed moods punctuated by frequent suicidal ideations. The initial treatment plan for San was merely targeted toward medication monitoring to stabilize San's mental status and functioning. Surprisingly, San did extremely well in the treatment milieu. She responded warmly to clients and staff, and the Program quickly became a surrogate family to her. San spent long hours daily at the Program, partaking first in ESL classes, and gradually moving into computer classes and formal VESID training. The attachment ties San developed with the Program were important to San's recovery and growth. Given San's familial circumstances–both her father and sister have built their own families–the Program filled an emotional void for her. The guidance and support from the staff, the camaraderie among the clients of similar age, and an ambience that fosters her bicultural identity as a young immigrant, provided San with a nurturing and stimulating environment. However, this did not preclude challenges and setbacks in San's course of recovery and growth, which in many ways paralleled the developmental phase of an adolescent. San's vocational training and convalescence in the Program was regularly disrupted by mini-crises brought on by San's impulsive decisions to take on demanding part-time jobs and pursuing romantic relationships.

The staff's acceptance of San's need for experimentation and individuation and San's reciprocal trust in the Program eventually sustained San's motivation in completing her vocational training and acquiring her GED. Around the same time, San also moved into her own apartment, which is part of CCC's Supportive Housing Program. San initially was torn between the obligations of her Asian self to care for her family and the wishes of her Western self to separate from her family. San and her social worker at CCC finally worked out a "compromise" that is culturally acceptable. With her social worker's assistance, San applied and got approval for increased SSI benefits. With careful budgeting, San was able to give her family a nominal sum of money each month to help defray their expenses. San also returned to her family on weekends to help her stepmother with household errands. San's assumption of the role of an adult child actually improved her relationship with her stepmother. San is now in the process of applying for a clerical job, and she continues to come to CCC for medication, socialization, and counseling.

Kee

Kee emigrated to the U.S. from the province of Fu Jian with his parents and three brothers at age sixteen. Kee is an extremely bright young man, and managed to master a good command of English within his two years in American high school. During his first year of college, Kee became withdrawn and depressed and eventually dropped out of college. Kee was hospitalized when his mental conditions deteriorated and he threatened to hurt his father and brothers. Kee was given a diagnosis of Bipolar Disorder, and he was referred to CCC for aftercare upon his discharge from the hospital. Kee was accompanied by his father at the intake session. Kee was mostly quiet and denied that he needed services. Kee's father, who was a restaurant worker, explained that he and two other sons mostly stayed in Maryland because of better employment opportunities, while his oldest son came home periodically on his days off from his restaurant in the suburbs of New York. In essence, Kee was left living with his mother who worked in a garment factory. It appeared that Kee was resentful that he had no choice in the family's emigration and resettlement plans.

Despite the earnestness of Kee's father to seek treatment and vocational training for his son at CCC, the intake staff team came up with a different plan to engage Kee. Kee was invited to visit the Program for a few days as a guest before he would have to decide whether he wanted to enroll in the Program. Kee eventually agreed to attend the Program for one hour three times a week. He kept a low profile for a long time, and declined to participate in any of the classes. He did slowly establish a relationship with his social worker who would call him when he did not show up at the Program as scheduled, and who provided assistance with his entitlements whenever needed.

After a year of sporadic attendance, Kee began to make some friends and spend more time socializing in the Program. He also confided more in his social worker regarding the conflicts he was having with his parents, especially his mother. Kee was resentful of his parents' pressure and expectations for him to return to work or school and support his mother while the rest of the family had basically "abandoned" the two of them.

At one point, Kee was having a great deal of arguments with his mother which greatly affected his moods and functioning. This occurred after Kee expressed his desire to move out of his mother's apartment and apply for one of the apartments under CCC's Supportive Housing Program. Kee vacillated between feeling confident and excited about living independently and fearful of leaving his mother alone and her angry and sad reactions. It appeared that Kee was faced with a cultural dilemma that could not be resolved without the sanction of his mother. Recognizing the severity of the stress for both Kee and his mother, CCC's administrator invited the two to attend a family session. Kee's mother was asked to speak about her life after the family immigrated to the U.S., which turned out to be a tale of poverty, poor housing, and the loss of family life. Apparently Kee's mother had been blamed by her husband and his extended family for Kee's mental illness, and she was not hopeful that her husband and other sons would be moving back. The staff validated her pain that she would be left with no family if Kee also moved out. Kee's mother cried as she felt understood, and she became less angry toward Kee. She acknowledged Kee's positive attributes and the progress he had made, and expressed appreciation for his loyalty to her. At the end of the interview, CCC's administrator pointed out the poignancy of how the staff's support of Kee's participation in the Program had undermined her closeness with Kee. Kee's mother, feeling emotionally stronger, came up with a "culturally compatible" response: "I want my son to succeed in life. As a mother, I have the obligation to help my son to succeed." This response was a powerful sanction of Kee's continued recovery. However, the emotionally charged issue of family closeness, which was highlighted in the session, was a cautionary note that Kee's recovery is very much tied to his mother's emotional recovery.

Kee has since resumed his socialization in the Program. His treatment goal consists of medication compliance and stabilization of his mental status. With fewer conflicts in the family, Kee has managed to achieve his treatment goal.

THE TRAGIC DISASTER OF SEPT. 11, 2001 AND ITS AFTERMATH

The spirit of CCC's therapeutic community could not have been more challenged by the tragic event that occurred on the morning of September 11, 2001. From the Lower East Side of Manhattan, CCC's staff and clients witnessed the two planes that crashed into the World Trade Center less than a mile away. Clients and staff held on to each other as they helplessly watched two landmark buildings collapse amidst screams, tears, and sirens. Shortly thereafter, a sea of people covered with soot and ashes ran into the neighborhood to seek refuge. On their own initiative, staff and clients set up tables and chairs on the sidewalk to offer refreshments and respite to the survivors. Some clients escorted those who needed to use the phones and bathrooms into the program facilities. Others attempted to comfort those who were emotionally distraught. Despite the initial shock and horror at the severity of the calamities, the clients appeared to be empowered by the experience. They continued to volunteer to staff a hospitality table outside the clinic the rest of the week. For the Chinese clients, the opportunity to support the larger community enhanced their feelings of being accepted in American society. It seemed that during the crisis many clients felt the need to be more connected to the Program and the therapeutic community. There were Chinese clients who lived in Brooklyn and Queens who braved the odds of disruptive subway services and continued to attend the Program the rest of the week to help out with chores. In subsequent discussions, some of the Chinese clients were able to share their previous experiences of violence and loss of loved ones in China, and relate their pain and fear to the feelings of the general community. While it is highly possible that there are delayed reactions to the tragedy, the majority of the clientele at CCC so far seems to be faring well. It appears that the Program has served as a safe haven for the clients during this difficult period, and the camaraderie that emerged in the therapeutic community has created a positive emotional experience for everyone.

TEACHING POINTS/DISCUSSION

CCC's Program Design and Philosophy

CCC's Day Treatment Program modality emphasizes a holistic view of the Chinese immigrant client in the context of his struggles to acculturate into a Western society, which are often hampered by the debilitating social and psychological effects of his mental illness. This view is reflected in CCC's program design, which aims at providing a positive acculturation milieu for the client as a vital component in his treatment plan. Two important and related aspects of acculturation are addressed in this milieu treatment: the immigrant client's adaptation to losses and the affirmation of his cultural heritage.

Adaptation to Losses

There are tremendous psychological losses associated with an individual's migration. These losses include one's kinship ties and social identity, as well as customs and rituals in one's cultural environment.

Leaving one's country involves profound loss. Often one has to give up familiar food, native music, unquestioned social customs, and even one's language. The new country offers strange-tasting food, new songs, different political concerns, unfamiliar language, pale festivals, unknown heroes, psychically unearned history, and a visually unfamiliar landscape. (Aktar, 1995, p. 1052)

It is generally agreed that the resolution of an immigrant's losses involves an integrative process of his identity, values and lifestyle from the immigrant's motherland and the new country (Aktar, 1995; Juthani, 1992; Meaders, 1997). This process entails the re-establishment of one's role within and outside the family, as well as the development of a sense of continuity and acceptance in the new environment.

In the case of CCC's Chinese clients who were unable to pursue gainful employment or education in this country because of their mental illness and the lack of vocational rehabilitation services, their adaptation process is severely curtailed. They received very little validation from their family and were isolated from society at large. In essence, there was a mounting sense of loss as they were cut off from both the old and the new worlds. Thus it is crucial that the first and foremost intervention strategy for these clients be targeted at counteracting their sense of powerlessness and loss, vis-à-vis the provision of a therapeutic milieu that supports the development of a bicultural identity.

Affirmation of the Immigrant's Cultural Heritage

As reflected in CCC's program design, acculturation for the immigrant client is a reciprocal process that validates the client's cultural heritage as well as facilitates his selection and adoption of new cultural values and norms. Meaders (1997) cautions the psychological risks of an immigrant who abandons his cultural heritage and embraces the dominant culture. Such devaluation of one's old culture and identity undermines one's sense of self, and increases one's vulnerability to being victimized by the undercurrents of society's racism. On the other hand, affirmation of an immigrant's cultural heritage affords the individual sanctions to accept one's original identity and ties as resources, from which one can complement with new values and lifestyles to form an expanded self.

A case in point is CCC's special efforts in soliciting the involvement of the Chinese clients' families in the treatment process. This is in recognition of the centrality of the family in the Asian culture, and support of the Asian sense of "collective self." The concerns of the client's family regarding economics and treatment are addressed, and the family is invited regularly to participate in counseling sessions and celebratory activities. As indicated earlier, sanctions from a client's family to seek treatment and adhere to the medication and rehabilitation regimen are crucial in expediting the client's recovery. In addition, the Chinese clients are encouraged to resolve their familial conflicts, and maintain their connections to the family throughout the treatment process. This intervention has proven to be effective in reinforcing the client's emotional stability, given the psychological significance of family ties in the Asian culture. At the same time, clients are also supported in their efforts to pursue individual vocational, educational and recreational interests. Thus, in essence, there is an integration of the Asian and western notion of "self." Instead of conformity versus individuation and separation, clients are encouraged to explore a more bicultural view of oneself as maintaining "connections" and "differentiation."

The Use of Asian Staff in a Multi-Cultural Treatment Team

A unique feature in CCC's program design is its use of Asian and non-Asian staff to create a multi-cultural milieu and a microcosm of American society. This is also a creative variation of cultural competent practice. As discussed earlier, the mix of Asian and non-Asian staff create enhanced feelings of acceptance and connection for the immigrant clients who are isolated from mainstream society. While the presence of Asian staff helps heal the immigrant clients' sense of loss, interaction with a multi-cultural staff that respects their cultural heritage is empowering and therapeutic in repairing their self-esteem.

IMPLICATIONS FOR PRACTICE

The program design of Community Consultation Center (CCC) is an effective treatment modality that can be replicated for any minority immigrant population that suffers from mental or physical disabilities. Its philosophy and service design support the social work values of acceptance of clients' differences and the maximization of their strengths vis-à-vis the provision of a nutritive environment. The integration of a diverse ethnic staff and client population is both a pragmatic and cost-effective way of service delivery.

REFERENCES

Akhtar, S. (1995). A third individuation: Immigration, identity, and the psychoanalytic process. *Journal of the American Psychoanalytic Association, 43*, 1051-1083.

Berry, J.W. (1984). Cultural relations in plural societies: Alternatives to segregation and their sociopsychological implications. In N. Miller & M. Brewer (Eds.), *Groups in contact* (pp. 11-27). New York: Academic Press.

Drachman, D. (1992). A stage-of-migration framework for service to immigrant populations. *Social Work, 37*, 68-72.

Greene, G. J., Jensen, C., & Jones, D. H. (1996). A constructivist perspective on clinical social work practice with ethnically diverse clients. *Social Work, 41*, 172-180.

Hsu, F. L. K. (1970) *Americans and Chinese*. New York: Doubleday.

Jacobson, N. (2001). Experiencing recovery: A dimensional analysis of recovery narratives. *Psychiatric Rehabilitation Journal, 24*, 248-255.

Juthani, N. (1992). Immigrant mental health: Conflicts and concerns of Indian immigrants in the U.S.A. *Psychology and Developing Societies, 4*, 133-148.

Kim, H. A. (1981). Mental health services for chronically mentally ill Asian Americans. In A. Ryan (Ed.), *Proceedings on Innovative Mental Health Services for Asian Americans* (pp. 20-21). New York, New York: Hunter College School of Social Work.

Lee, E. (1996). Asian American Families. In M. McGoldrick, J. Giordano, & J. Pearce (Eds.), *Ethnicity and Family Therapy, 2nd Edition* (pp. 249-267). New York: Guilford Press.

Meaders, N.Y. (1997). The transcultural self. In P. Ellowitz, & C. Kahn (Eds.), *Immigrant experiences, personal narratives and psychological analyses* (pp. 47-59). Cranberry, NJ: Associated University Press.

McNeil, J. S., & Kennedy, R. (1997). Mental health services to minority groups of color. In T.R. Watkins, & J. W. Callicutt (Eds.), *Mental health policy and practice today* (pp. 235-257). Thousand Oaks, California: Sage Publications.

Owan, T. C. (1981). Neighborhood based mental health: An approach to overcome inequalities in mental health services delivery to racial and ethnic minorities. In A. Ryan (Ed.), *Proceedings on Innovative Mental Health Services for Asian Americans* (pp. 42-43). New York, New York: Hunter College School of Social Work.

Roland, A. (1994). Identity, self, and individualism in a multicultural perspective. In E. P. Salett, & D.R. Koslow (Eds.), *Race, Ethnicity, and Self* (pp. 11-23). Wash. D.C.: NMCI Publications.

Ross-Sheriff, F. (1992). Adaptation and integration into American society: Major issues affecting Asian Americans. In S. M. Furuto, R. Biswas, D. Chung, K. Murase, F. Ross-Sheriff (Eds.), *Social Work Practice with Asian Americans* (pp. 45-63). Newbury Park: Sage Publications.

Saleeby, D. (1996). The strengths perspective in social work practice: Extensions and cautions. *Social Work, 41*, 296-305.

Sue, S., & Morishima, J. (1982). *The Mental Health of Asian Americans*. San Francisco: Jossey-Bass, Inc.

Uba, L. (1994). *Asian Americans: Personality Patterns, Identity, and Mental Health*. New York, New York: The Guilford Press.

Winnicott, D.W. (1965). *The Maturational Processes and the Facilitating Environment*. Madison, Connecticut: International Universities Press, Inc.

Wong, H. (1981). Individual, group, and system considerations in the mental health treatment of chronically ill Asian Americans. In A. Ryan (Ed.), *Proceedings on Innovative Mental Health Services for Asian Americans* (pp. 49-53). New York, New York: Hunter College School of Social Work.

Conclusion

Diane Drachman
Ana Paulino

SUMMARY. This Conclusion discusses ideas that evolve out of the work presented in this volume; raises issues and questions for further study; and reconfigures previous work on the migration process. *[Article copies available for a fee from The Haworth Document Delivery Service: 1-800-HAWORTH. E-mail address: <docdelivery@haworthpress.com> Website: <http://www.HaworthPress.com> © 2004 by The Haworth Press, Inc. All rights reserved.]*

KEYWORDS. Social work, immigration, undocumented immigrants, return migration, circular migration

The volume includes discussions on different types of immigrant groups: transnational, circular, return and undocumented. These different groups encounter unique experiences which require identification and greater understanding in order to adequately provide services to them.

Diane Drachman, PhD, is Associate Professor, University of Connecticut School of Social Work.

Ana Paulino, EdD, is Associate Professor and Chair, Children, Youth, and Families Field of Practice/Specialization, Hunter College School of Social Work.

[Haworth co-indexing entry note]: "Conclusion." Drachman, Diane, and Ana Paulino. Co-published simultaneously in *Journal of Immigrant & Refugee Services* (The Haworth Social Work Practice Press, an imprint of The Haworth Press) Vol. 2, No. 1/2, 2004, pp. 161-171; and: *Immigrants and Social Work: Thinking Beyond the Borders of the United States* (ed: Diane Drachman, and Ana Paulino) The Haworth Social Work Practice Press, an imprint of The Haworth Press, Inc., 2004, pp. 161-171. Single or multiple copies of this article are available for a fee from The Haworth Document Delivery Service [1-800-HAWORTH, 9:00 a.m. - 5:00 p.m. (EST). E-mail address: docdelivery@haworthpress.com].

http://www.haworthpress.com/web/JIRS
© 2004 by The Haworth Press, Inc. All rights reserved.
Digital Object Identifier: 10.1300/J191v02n01_10

As identified by Dr. Healy, family re-unification is a special concern for the transnational family. An understanding of family reunification however, includes examination of the experiences in both sending and receiving countries. For example, in Jamaica, social workers in contact with children who are separated from parents who have migrated to another country cite the sense of abandonment experienced by some children. Also for some, child care arrangements are either unsuitable or fail. Social workers in the United States (U.S.), on the other hand, observe the difficulty in re-building relationships when families re-unify due in part to the long separation.

Complexity is added when family reunification occurs in the context of a different family structure. For example, a spouse or companion could be added to the family living in the new country of residence. Other children could be born. Step and/or half brothers and sisters could be added. Thus, the child who remained in the home country and reunites with the family enters into a different family form. The incorporation of the reunified child into the family also means the family structure is changed for other members. Therefore, all members have to adjust or re-adjust to one another (Drachman, Kwon-Ahn, & Paulino, 1996).

Children and parents may hold different views on migration. As cited by Dr. Healy, children commonly experience their parents' migration as abandonment. On the other hand, parents often view their migration as providing a better life and greater opportunity for their children (Drachman, Kwon-Ahn, & Paulino, 1996). The dissensus in views can lead to family conflict. Some parents view the child as ungrateful given the sacrifices made on the child's behalf. Others feel guilty upon learning that the child care arrangements in the home country were problematic. The additive affects of initial separation from the parent(s), a problematic caretaking arrangement in the home country and the upheaval of a recent migration lead some children to resent their parents and other family members (Drachman, Kwon-Ahn, & Paulino, 1996). The behavioral expressions of the above issues vary and include school difficulties and acting out behavior among some children, persistent conflict among siblings, conflict between parents and children, and scapegoating of the re-unified child who is often viewed as the cause of the family's problems (Drachman, Kwon-Ahn, & Paulino, 1996).

Members of the transnational family (frequently parents) also return to the home country. Thus, family reunification occurs in reverse migration. As Dr. Healy suggests, cross national collaboration between ser-

vice personnel in sending and receiving countries could provide information on family reunification as it occurs in both countries. The sharing
of information accumulated in each of the countries could establish a
beginning and broad context for understanding this aspect of the transnational family.

The traumatic realities associated with the immigration of undocumented Mexican immigrants are clearly portrayed by Dr. Zuniga. Their
life threatening experiences in the home country, their experiences of
abuse in the new country, and the families who witness the death of a
family member during the immigration journey provide a context for
understanding the mental health issues experienced by some persons in
this population.

Dr. Zuniga also discusses the current anti-immigrant social climate in
the U.S. Among the examples cited are California's proposition 187
which sought to deny undocumented residents from receiving welfare
and educational benefits. Other examples cited include two 1996 legislative acts–the Illegal Immigration Reform and Immigrant Responsibility Act (IIRIRA) and the Personal Responsibility and Work Opportunity Reconciliation Act (PRWORA). As its title suggests, the IIRIRA is
aimed at curbing the immigration of persons without authorization to
enter the country. Both laws, however, are aimed at all immigrant
groups. Combined, these laws curb immigrants rights, reduce their eligibility for services and require federally-funded welfare organizations
to report information on immigrant clients to the Bureau of Immigration &
Customs Service–previously the Immigration & Naturalization Service.

As a counterpoint to the above, Dr. Zuniga cites the 2001 California legislation which permits undocumented immigrant students to pay college
tuition fees at the more economical state resident rate vs. the expensive out
of state resident fee. Thus, a pro-immigrant rights and humanitarian force
concurrently occurs within an anti-immigrant climate.

Competing concurrent forces have historically influenced immigration debates, legislation and policy. Underlying these forces are foreign
policy issues, economics, racism, xenophobia, anti-ethnic sentiments,
civil rights, and humanitarianism (Drachman & Ryan, 2001). Economic
forces are currently driving the recognition and acceptance of an identity card known as the matricula card. This card is issued by the
Mexican government to all Mexican immigrants including undocumented Mexican nationals. The card has enabled the undocumented
Mexican immigrant population to borrow books from the library, to apply for
a permit to operate a vending cart, to open a bank account, receive a debit

card and to present it to police who accept the card from crime victims (Swarns, 2003).

According to some officials in the Midwest, the card will be a boon to local economies, encouraging Mexican immigrants to pour money into banks and businesses. Since Mexican workers are increasingly filling jobs in small towns, their needs can not be ignored; and recognition of the matricula card is simply a reflection of the changes rippling across the Midwest (Swarns, 2003).

A foreign policy issue also underlies the acceptance of the card. After the September 11th terrorist attacks on the U.S., the discussions between Mexico and the U.S. on amnesty for Mexican undocumented immigrants living in the U.S. were derailed. As a result, Mexican diplomats began lobbying throughout the U.S. for the card's acceptance. Currently, many cities, states, police departments and financial institutions accept the card (Swarns, 2003).

The rising death rate among Mexican and Central Americans during their perilous journey "north" has led some U.S. legislators to introduce bills that would grant these migrants legal but temporary guest worker entry into the U.S. (Padgett, 2003). Thus, a humanitarian force is currently apparent.

Concern for the civil rights of immigrants is also developing momentum and countering anti immigrant forces. For example, labor unions, foundations, churches and civil rights groups sponsored a cross country bus ride to persuade Congress and the public to support legislation which would provide legal status for millions of undocumented immigrants in the U.S. (Greenhouse, 2003). Other goals of the ride included: providing full labor protections for undocumented workers; respecting the civil rights of all immigrant workers including the undocumented; and expanding family reunification visas for relatives of legal immigrants (Greenhouse, 2003).

This advocacy effort was an unprecedented mobilization in support of immigrants in this country. The bus riders stopped for rallies in dozens of cities. In Tucson, they commemorated the deaths of immigrants who died in the desert during their immigration trek. Finally, they met other bus riders in Washington, D.C. to rally and lobby for immigrants' rights.

Attitudes toward immigration and immigrants have had historic swings between inclusion and exclusion. The competing forces noted above underlie the attitudinal swings. In the context of an anti-immigrant climate, the forces for civil rights and humanitarianism can be joined. Furthermore, they can coalesce with other supporting forces such as the foreign policy and economic issues that are driving acceptance of the matricula card and leading legislators to introduce bills for immigrants' safety and rights. The joining of forces can strengthen the position for inclusion. Social workers' awareness and familiarity with these historic/ present and often concurrent forces can facilitate thinking of ways to advocate and coalesce with others in support of the needs and rights of immigrant populations.

The return of immigrants from the U.S. to their native country is both an historic and current phenomenon. Reverse or return migration also occurs in other countries with immigrant populations. As Dr. Guzzetta states, return migration is as old as migration itself. In his discussion, Dr. Guzzetta raises the issue of the limited data gathering by the U.S. on reverse migration despite the sizeable amount and quite reliable demographic information on arrivals. The lack of systematic data collection on returnees ultimately leads to broad and conflicting estimates. For example, the Social Security Administration assumes one-third of all U.S. immigrants emigrate while the I.N.S. estimates return migration falls between 20-25%. As Dr. Guzzetta indicates, discussions of the current needs of populations, proposals for services, and predictions of future needs are dependent on reliable data.

The limited attention paid to return migration has also contributed to limited analysis of the types of return migrants and the experiences associated with the types. We know that transnational immigrants return to their home country for short or long stays. Some return for a year or several years and then return to the U.S. The variable of age at the time of return and subsequent return to the U.S. is likely to influence the nature of the return experiences. The duration of the return(s) each way could influence the experience. The experience may also be different if an individual returns by him/herself vs. a return with family members.

The back and forth movement among Puerto Ricans between the island and the U.S. mainland is discussed by Dr. Acevedo under the concept of circular migration. A return to the homeland is obviously embedded in the circular pattern. Circular migration, according to Dr. Acevedo, is perceived by some analysts of the pattern as dysfunctional for children's education and family life. Dr. Acevedo, however, interprets circular migration as an adaptive and flexible response to globalization and to social and economic problems that exist on both the island and mainland.

Transnational and circular immigrants comprise a growing section of immigrant families in the U.S. As discussed in the immigration and transnational literatures, their evolution and growth are responses to macro forces of economics, social, political, and technological changes. However, knowledge of the strategies transnational and Puerto Rican circular migrants utilize to manage their individual and family lives in the context of back and forth movements, or to overcome obstacles associated with the returns, and finally, to adapt would also provide needed information for social workers practicing in family service, child welfare, community, and mental health settings. This is another area for cross national study in sending and receiving countries.

The discussion of Dominican migration to the U.S. by Dr. Hernández focuses on the interconnectedness of large systemic forces in both sending and receiving countries. The influence of transforming economies in the Dominican Republic and in the U.S. at different time periods are examined. External and internal pressures in the Dominican Republic aimed at population reduction (based on a belief that poverty is the result of procreation); economic growth concurrent with high levels of unemployment; a pressure to eliminate dissidents; and U.S. interest in maintaining stability in the country are among the historical systemic factors underlying the migration of Dominicans to the U.S. The U.S. legislative changes in immigration during the 1980s and 1990s with their emphasis on "exclusion" and "closing doors" have resulted in the deportation of many Dominicans and fewer arrivals from the Dominican Republic. Dr. Hernández's longitudinal historical analysis sheds light on the changes in each of the countries over time and the consequences of these changes for Dominican immigrants. Thus, a broad context for understanding Dominican migration to the U.S. emerges.

Immigrants commonly struggle with the discrepancy between their expectations for life in a new land and the reality of the experiences they encounter in the new country of residence (Drachman, 1992; Drachman, Kwon-Ahn, & Paulino, 1996; Drachman & Ryan, 2001). The ways in which this common immigrant experience are uniquely expressed in the lives of low income Mexican women are illustrated in the qualitative research of Drs. Marquez and Padilla. The women in the study migrated for economic reasons. They settled in either the northern border of Mexico or in the U.S. at the Mexican border. The women living in Mexico were able to find work. However, the high cost of living at the border offset their wages which ultimately sustained a life of poverty. Their "work lives" were also shortened as women who were pregnant were fired; and women 30 and over could not find work. Women living at the U.S. border could also find work. Their low wages, undocumented immigration status, limited education and gender-segregated jobs also sustained a life of poverty. Despite the disjuncture between their expectations for a better economic life and the reality of the economic struggles in the new region/country, the survival strategies of the women in the context of families, households and migration emerge. The depth and importance of cultural phenomena as they relate to migration are portrayed in two distinctly different papers: Drs. Humphreys and Haroutunian's "Armenian Refugees and Displaced Persons and the Birth of Armenian Social Work"; and Dr. Chung and Ms. Samperi's "An East-West Approach to Serving Chinese Immigrants in a Mental Health Setting." Each paper serves as a model for its unique work.

Despite the experience of genocide, forced migration, and dispersal throughout the world, Armenians from the diaspora returned to the new Republic of Armenia to assist earthquake survivors in the country. Their return to the country reflects the depth of their cultural attachment to their people and their land. As Drs. Humphreys and Haroutunian note, many Armenians in the diaspora had never been to Armenia. However, the people and the country had been kept alive in their minds through the stories told to them by their parents and grandparents. Their voluntary assistance and economic contributions at the time and currently has had enormous benefit for the nation and its people. The birth of social work in Armenia is in part the result of their contributions.

Although the discussion of Drs. Humphreys and Haroutunian covers the Armenian diaspora and the migration of refugees and displaced persons following the fall of the Soviet Union, the description of the cross national social work activity is unique as it provides social workers with a model for this type work. The cross national activities have resulted in the development of the first school of social work in Armenia including the development of field work sites. Exchanges between social work faculties and students in Armenia and the U.S. have taken place. Furthermore, courses have been simultaneously delivered to Armenian and U.S. social work students through electronic media. The work is an ongoing binational product.

Dr. Chung and Ms. Samperi's discussion portrays the ways in which cultural meanings regarding immigration, emotional disturbance, work, family, customs and rituals held by Chinese immigrants are embodied in the procedures and services offered to this population in a multi cultural community mental health setting. For example, intake procedures are provided by Chinese bicultural service providers. The client's family is engaged at intake in recognition of its importance in Chinese cultural life. The significance attached to work by Chinese clients is recognized by incorporating vocational services and skills training into the helping plans. Chinese holidays are celebrated. Chinese clients develop their own theatre productions and Chinese food is served in the day treatment program.

Concurrently, Chinese clients are introduced to U.S. multicultural populations who are also served at the day treatment program. Their beliefs, customs, holidays, food, and theatre productions are also incorporated into the varied services of the program. Service providers and staff are multiethnic, racially diverse, and represent the mix of different populations in the U.S.

The program serves as a model for the management of mental illness in the context of immigration and Chinese culture while concurrently familiarizing "newcomers" to U.S. society, its cultural and racial mix of people, its institutions, and its customs.

Finally, the work of the authors in this volume has generated a revision in thinking about the migration process. In previous work, the migration experience is conceptualized in phases and formulated in a framework on stages of migration (Drachman, 1990, 1992; Drachman & Halberstadt, 1992; Drachman, Kwon-Ahn, & Paulino 1996; Drachman & Ryan, 2001). The framework provides a context for understanding and helping immigrants and refugees by linking the migration experiences that occur in the country of origin with experiences that occur in an intermediate country and finally with the experiences in the country of destination. Since service personnel are not in contact with "newcomers" until they arrive in the country of destination, the framework offers a way for workers to consider *the intermingling* between migration experiences in the home country and the intermediate country with the resettlement experiences in the U.S. The cumulative effect of experiences and movements in the migration process also becomes more apparent.

The framework is conceptualized in three stages–pre-migration/departure, transit/intermediate, and resettlement. The diagram in Table 1 outlines the stages of migration, the critical variables associated with each stage, and common factors that influence each migration stage (Drachman, 1992).

For some immigrant populations, the framework is useful. Its application has been useful in understanding varied immigrant groups including Southeast Asians (O & Porr, 1990); Haitians (DeWind, 1990); Cubans (Gil, 1990); Russians (Mandel, 1990; Drachman & Halberstadt, 1992; Drachman & Ryan, 2001); Koreans (Drachman, Kwon-Ahn, & Paulino, 1996); and Dominicans (Drachman, Kwon Ahn & Paulino, 1996). However, the discussions in this volume on transnational, circular, and return migrants indicate that for some immigrant groups, the migration process does not end with resettlement

TABLE 1. Stage of Migration Framework

Stage of Migration	Critical Variables	Factors That Influence Each Migration Stage
Premigration	Social, political, economic and educational factors Separation from family and friends Decisions about who leaves and who is left behind Abrupt departure Long wait and living in limbo prior to departure Leaving a familiar environment Life-threatening circumstances Experiences of violence and/or persecution Loss of significant others	Age Family composition
Transit/Intermediate	Perilous or safe journey of short or long duration Refugee camp or detention center stay of short or long duration Awaiting a foreign country's decision regarding final relocation Loss of significant others	Urban/rural background Education Culture Socioeconomic background Occupation Belief system Social support
Resettlement	Cultural issues Reception from host country Opportunity structure of host country Discrepancy between expectations and reality Degree of cumulative stress throughout migration process Different levels of acculturation among family members	

as formulated in the above framework. For some, the migration process involves back and forth movements between the country of origin and destination; or migration to a third country and a return to the home country or a return to the previous receiving country. The pattern of movements can vary. The diagram in the Appendix expands the formulation of the migration process and takes into account both migration that ends at resettlement and migration that extends beyond resettlement. However, the critical factors associated with the return(s) to the country of origin and subsequent return(s) to the receiving country, or migration to a third country and return to the receiving or sending country are largely unknown at this time. Knowledge of these factors are likely to evolve out of cross national studies and further research in this area.

REFERENCES

DeWind, J. (1990). Haitian boat people in the United States: Background for social service providers. In D. Drachman (Ed.), *Social services to refugee populations* (pp. 7-56). Washington, DC: National Institute of Mental Health.

Drachman, D. (1990). *Social services to refugee populations*. Washington, DC: National Institute of Mental Health.

Drachman, D. (1992). A stage of migration framework for services to immigrant populations. *Social Work*, 37, 68-72.

Drachman, D., & Halberstadt, A. (1992). Stage of migration framework as applied to recent Soviet emigres. In A.S. Ryan (Ed.), *Social work with immigrants and refugees*. New York: The Haworth Press, Inc.

Drachman, D., Y.H. Kwon-Ahn, & A. Paulino (1996). Migration and resettlement experiences of Dominican and Korean families. *Families in Society* 77(10): 626-38.

Drachman, D., & Ryan, A.S. (2001). Immigrants and refugees. In A. Gitterman (Ed.) *Handbook of social work with vulnerable and resilient populations.*

Gil, R. (1990). Cuban refugees: Implications for clinical social work practice. In D. Drachman (Ed.) *Social services to refugee populations* (pp. 57-72). Washington, DC: National Institute of Mental Health.

Greenhouse, S. (2003). Riding across America for immigrant workers. *New York Times*, September 17, p. A20.

Lichtblau, E. (2003). U.S. report faults the roundup of illegal immigrants after 9/11. *New York Times*, June 3, PA1.

Mandel, L. (1990). Soviet refugees. In D. Drachman (Ed.) *Social services to refugee populations* (pp. 79-90). Washington, DC: National Institute of Mental Health.

O, S.L., & Porr, P. (1990). Social work practice with Indochinese refugees. In D. Drachman (Ed.), *Social service to refugee populations* (pp. 91-120). Washington, DC: National Institute of Mental Health.

Padgett, T. (2003). People smugglers inc. *Time*, August 18, pp. 42-44.

Swarns, Rachel (2003). Old ID cards give new status to Mexicans in the U.S. *New York Times*, August 25, PA1.

APPENDIX. Stages of Migration: Critical Variables

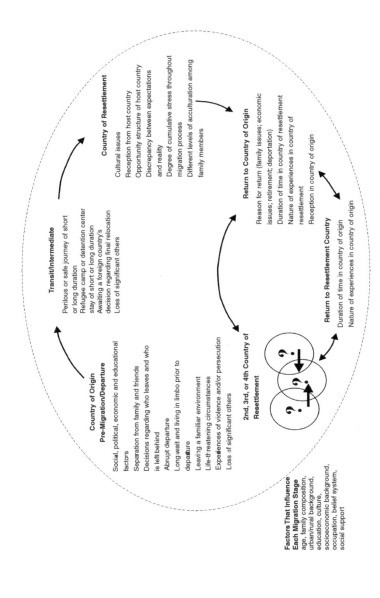

**Country of Origin
Pre-Migration/Departure**

Social, political, economic and educational factors

Separation from family and friends

Decisions regarding who leaves and who is left behind

Abrupt departure

Long wait and living in limbo prior to departure

Leaving a familiar environment

Life-threatening circumstances

Experiences of violence and/or persecution

Loss of significant others

Transit/Intermediate

Perilous or safe journey of short or long duration

Refugee camp or detention center stay of short or long duration

Awaiting a foreign country's decision regarding final relocation

Loss of significant others

Country of Resettlement

Cultural issues

Reception from host country

Opportunity structure of host country

Discrepancy between expectations and reality

Degree of cumulative stress throughout migration process

Different levels of acculturation among family members

2nd, 3rd, or 4th Country of Resettlement

Return to Resettlement Country

Duration of time in country of origin

Nature of experiences in country of origin

Return to Country of Origin

Reason for return (family issues; economic issues; retirement; deportation)

Duration of time in country of resettlement

Nature of experiences in country of resettlement

Reception in country of origin

Factors That Influence Each Migration Stage

age, family composition, urban/rural background, education, culture, socioeconomic background, occupation, belief system, social support

171

Index

T - #0246 - 101024 - C0 - 212/152/10 [12] - CB - 9780789019981 - Gloss Lamination